The Denial of Aging

The Denial of Aging

*Perpetual Youth, Eternal Life,
and Other Dangerous
Fantasies*

MURIEL R. GILLICK, M.D.

HARVARD UNIVERSITY PRESS
Cambridge, Massachusetts
London, England
2006

Library of Congress Cataloging-in-Publication Data

Gillick, Muriel R., 1951–
The denial of aging : perpetual youth, eternal life,
and other dangerous fantasies / Muriel R. Gillick.
p. cm.
ISBN 0-674-02148-7 (alk. paper)
1. Old age—United States.
2. Old age—United States—Planning.
3. Older people—United States.
4. Aging—United States.
5. Retirement—United States.   I. Title.
HQ1064.U5G45 2006
646.7'9'0973—dc22   2005052546

Designed by Gwen Nefsky Frankfeldt

In memory of Anne Coates,
who knew all about a good old age
but did not live to have one

Contents

Prelude   *1*

1. An Ounce of Prevention?   *11*

2. When Less Is More   *37*

3. Doing the Right Thing Near the End   *63*

4. The Trouble with Medicare   *93*

5. Is a Nursing Home in Your Future?   *123*

6. Assisted Living: Boon or Boondoggle?   *159*

7. The Lure of Immortality   *195*

8. Making the Most of the Retirement Years   *225*

   Finale   *255*

   Appendix: Resources and References   *273*
   Notes   *289*
   Acknowledgments   *331*
   Index   *333*

The Denial of Aging

Prelude

Along with photographs of his wife, children, and grandchildren, Eric Braun kept a striking picture of himself as a young man.[1] He had evidently been a body-builder, long before pumping iron was the vogue. The picture featured my patient wearing tight-fitting bathing trunks and nothing else, flexing his generous arm muscles, and beaming. This was a man who had done everything right: he had studied hard and been successful in school, propelling himself out of urban squalor to the City University of New York and from there to medical school. During all his years of medical training, as an intern, a resident, and then a fellow specializing in allergy, he ran a minimum of a mile a day. He lifted weights. He ate a low-fat, low-cholesterol diet with plenty of fiber, resisting the temptations of ice cream sundaes, beer, and chips which served as the respective indulgences of his family, fellow physicians, and children. He exercised his mind along with his body: he was an avid reader and continued to practice medicine until the age of 78, when he had his first stroke.

When I first met Dr. Braun, he was in his eighties and he had had several additional strokes. The net effect was that he was virtually paralyzed—he could not lift his hand to scratch an itch or dial a phone number. His legs were so weak that he needed help to roll over in bed. His balance was so poor that when he sat in a chair, which he could not do for long periods because his back and neck got sore, he had to be propped up with pillows and literally held in place with a lap belt.

Following his first stroke but before the latest, Dr. Braun had lived at home with 24-hour caregivers. Initially, he had a single live-in assistant who had her own room and whose services were needed to help him get up in the morning, prepare his meals, and put him to bed at night. After the second stroke, it took two people to get him to a chair or the toilet, so he hired a second live-in aide. But he began waking up during the night and requiring assistance, disrupting the sleep of his helpers. His family decided that the best approach was to have multiple caregiving shifts throughout the day. After his third stroke, he had two nurse's aides for each of three 8-hour shifts, seven days a week. The burn rate for this living arrangement was phenomenal. After a few months, he moved to a nursing home and I became his physician.

Dr. Braun had been an extraordinary man. His daughter assured me that in addition to being a superb physician and a devoted husband, he was a wonderful father. He gave money to charity. He even had a sense of humor. He did not drink or smoke. And yet he lived for five years in a state that he increasingly viewed as intolerable. He was more dependent than an infant—and considerably more difficult for others to bathe or dress because they could not simply pick him up—and he was excruciatingly aware of his situation.

Perhaps if Dr. Braun had not exercised and eaten well, he would have had his strokes ten years earlier. As shown by the story of Jim Fixx, the marathoner who died of a heart attack at age 52, life-style change can only go so far in counterbalancing genetic predisposition. We would like to think that if we eat nutritious meals and exercise faithfully, we will be able to fend off old age. When we believe we will stay young forever, and when we purchase special vitamins, herbs, and other youth-enhancing chemicals to promote longevity, we are engaging in massive denial.

Americans spend an extraordinary $6 billion each year on "anti-aging" nostrums. Both the baby boomers and older people swallow pills and dietary supplements that purport to prevent illness, cure disease, and promote long life. The industry is largely unregulated, which led one senator, the chair of the Senate Special Committee on Aging, to initiate a probe of anti-aging scams. His investigation produced overwhelming evidence that the potions are ineffective at best, harmful at worst—and a phenomenal waste of money overall.[2]

We also spend an exorbitant amount of money covering up the stigmata of old age. The use of hair color is so ubiquitous that I could not find any estimates of the amount of money spent on vanquishing the gray. Botox injections to eliminate wrinkles are a recent addition to the youth-promoting armamentarium. Botox joins the facelift, a major surgical procedure to reduce wrinkles, and liposuction, a surgical fix for fat, in the growing list of mechanical techniques for hiding aging.

The expenditure on anti-aging books is modest in comparison to the outlay on pills and injections, but it is striking that the number of books purporting to prevent aging far surpasses those that address coping with aging. A visit to the library, the bookstore, or any online bookseller reveals titles such as *Grow Younger, Live Longer: 10 Steps to Reverse Aging* and *Stop Aging Now! The Ultimate Plan for Staying Young and Reversing the Aging Process.* Readers are exhorted to "defy" aging.[3] A visit to the search engine Google resulted in 227,000 hits when I typed in "anti-aging." But as the leader of an effort to debunk the anti-aging rhetoric put it, claims that we can slow, stop, or reverse aging have been made for thousands of years, and "they are as false today as they were in the past."[4]

Contemporary Americans are eager to prevent, obliterate, or at least conceal old age and, in keeping with the belief that we can control our destiny, we believe we will succeed. But the obsession with youth has not always prevailed, though there have always been seekers of immortality. America in the immediate post–Revolutionary War period was decidedly gerontophilic. In the seventeenth century, wigs were fashionable for men, powdered white because people *wanted* to look old. The seating in New England meetinghouses in the same period reflected the status of the old—the best seats were reserved for them.[5] While there is some degree of controversy about exactly when veneration metamorphosed into disdain, the consensus is that by 1820 the transformation was complete. Subsequent laws and regulations created clearer demarcations between old and young. Social Security and later Medicare were beneficial in providing much-needed assistance for the old, but they also served to further divide the population into productive youths and superannuated elders.

The final decades of the twentieth century brought a resurgence of interest in positive aging. Betty Friedan, in her book *The Fountain of Age*, advocated a second career for retirees,[6] and *Modern Maturity*, the magazine of the American Association of Retired Persons (now called *AARP: The Magazine*), featured the image of the golf-playing, globe-trotting senior flourishing in an upscale condominium complex. While acknowledgment of the possibilities of old age is laudable, the new breed of gerontophiles recognizes only one type of old age, one that is marked by vigor and good health. Friedan, in fact, goes so far as to deny that Alzheimer's disease actually exists. She attributes confusion and disorientation in the elderly exclusively to the effects of medication or premature institutionalization.

The reality is that very advanced age is in the cards for many of us: life expectancy at age 65 is 19.2 years for American women and 15.9 years for American men.[7] At least some of those years are likely to be marred by physical debility, cognitive impairment, or both. Moreover, there will be a great many older people in the coming decades. In the year 2030 there will be 70 million people in America over the age of 65, including 8.5 million people over the age of 85. We know this with reasonable certainty because these people are already alive today. Unless there is a major deterioration in public health (as happened in Russia) or a new plague (like AIDS, but principally affecting the old), we can predict with confidence how many people will survive to old age. The enormous increase in the number of elders, particularly the oldest old, will create a variety of challenges. These challenges will be triggered in part by the costs associated with extending our current approach to medical care to this larger population, and also by the need to find caregivers for the millions of people who will require help with the most basic activities of daily life. And the sheer numbers will push us to ask a question that in the past we have largely shied away from, insisting it's all a matter of personal choice: What is the *right* approach to medical care for those near the end of life?

Instead of tackling these difficult questions, we have chosen to engage in collective denial of aging. We would prefer to believe that most people can skip old age altogether—proceeding directly from middle age (itself an extension of youth) to death, preferably dying in one's sleep. We put our faith in exercise and diet as a means of assuring a healthy and vigorous old age, even though many of the principal scourges of old age cannot be prevented through exercise or diet.

Denial is sometimes a good thing: it can help us cope with intolerable truths. In the case of aging, however, widespread belief in perpetual youth or eternal life has pernicious consequences. If we as a society continue to deny the realities of old age, we will squander our resources on ineffective but costly screening tests and on ultimately futile but expensive treatment near the end of life; we will not have enough money left over to provide beneficial care. If we assume that Alzheimer's disease will be cured and disability abolished in the near term, we will have no incentive to develop long-term-care facilities that focus on enabling residents to lead satisfying lives despite their disabilities. If we assume that diet and exercise will prevent chronic disease, then we will fail to take seriously the need for a radically new model of medical care that is up to the task of caring for patients with chronic illness. We will not bother to institute a major overhaul of the Medicare program that incorporates the new model. And if we put our faith in drugs to make us immortal, we will neglect to fund research into such prosaic conditions as macular degeneration (the leading cause of visual impairment in the American elderly) and osteoarthritis (the number one medical problem in the elderly and a major source of pain and immobility), disorders that impair the quality of life of millions.

At the same time, we need to appreciate that older people are not a homogeneous group. They include robust elders, people who are independent and vigorous, though they may carry various diagnoses and need to take assorted pills to stay healthy. They encompass the frail elderly, individuals who typically have multiple interacting disorders, problems that together conspire to make them dependent in some of their most basic functions such as bathing or dressing. Frail people have limited reserves—their heart, lungs, and kidneys may work well enough to permit them to get by day to day, but a fairly minor stress such as a respiratory infection or sometimes a new medication can push them over the edge into severe illness. The elderly also include those with dementia, a constellation of diagnoses including Alzheimer's disease, vascular dementia, and other conditions with names like

Lewy Body disease and Pick's disease, all of which are progressive and ultimately fatal. People with dementia need help getting by in the world: they need assistance with cooking and shopping as well as with more fundamental activities such as using the bathroom. They are often unsafe if unsupervised and, like frail elders, they are fragile—vulnerable to even greater degrees of confusion with minimal provocation. Among the elderly are those who have both frailty and dementia, whose bodies and minds are equally impaired. This group has all the problems of the frail plus the needs of the demented. And finally, the elderly include those who are at the very end of their lives, who are expected to die within months, regardless of how much medical treatment they receive.[8]

Recognizing the variety of health statuses among the elderly is crucial because underlying health is an important determinant of people's needs. Preferences are critical—people have different pain thresholds, as well as varying tolerance for discomfort or uncertainty or disability. Preferences are shaped to a great extent by values, which in turn reflect ethnicity and religion as well as personality. But preferences are also shaped by physical reality, and thus an understanding of prognosis and possibility is as essential as culture and class in deciding how much medical care and what kind make sense for a given person.

A good old age involves more than physical health. At least as important as health is an individual's emotional, spiritual, and social life. Also critical is the environment, the home and community in which a person lives. And the ultimate determinant of a good old age is the ability to derive meaning from life, with all the other factors (health, emotional well-being, housing, and so on) serving to facilitate a sense of purpose, belonging, and continuity.[9]

In this book I try to lay the groundwork for a satisfying old age by looking at some of the most important areas affecting each group of elders—their health care, where they live, and how they find meaning in their lives. For each segment of the elderly population—the robust, the frail, and the dying—I will ask what is right and what is wrong with the current approach. Through the stories of my patients and my family, who run the gamut from the robust to the dying, some answers will begin to emerge.

The good news is that America has the know-how, the resources, and the imagination needed to adequately and appropriately provide for our seniors. But we need to act now to be sure that the necessary changes will be implemented by the time the baby boomers reach old age. We need to change patients' expectations of physicians, particularly in the area of health prevention and health maintenance, to better conform to what we have learned from evidence-based medicine. We need to modify physicians' behavior to ensure that older patients are treated in accordance with geriatric principles. All of us—physicians, patients, and relatives—have to learn when it's time to stop. The Medicare program must be substantially overhauled, not merely expanded to provide comprehensive prescription drug coverage, in order to meet the needs of those with chronic illness. Nursing homes, which currently house 1.6 million people and which will continue to provide care for the neediest and most disabled elders, have to be transformed from institutions into homes. Assisted living, in principle an ideal way to balance the need for care and the desire for autonomy in old age, will have to be revamped to fulfill its promise. The scientific research agenda must be focused on the problems that affect the quality of life of older people. And we should work on developing the kind of society—more communitarian and less individualistic—that will allow older people to flourish. Once we abandon the myths of perpetual youth and eternal life, we can do the exciting work described in this book—and get ready for old age.

ONE

An Ounce of Prevention?

Ever since Everett Koop catapulted the office of the Surgeon-General to national prominence, the American public has turned to the Surgeon-General for health advice. And the advice we have been getting since the publication of the report *Healthy People* has been that we need to take responsibility for our health.[1] The secret weapon against illness is prevention: more women should get annual mammograms; more people should wear seatbelts; more people should quit smoking. In general, American medicine focuses far too heavily on heroic rescues of patients with advanced diseases and attends much too little to prevention. The drumroll for "health maintenance" has had to be loud to compete with the brassy calls for invasive and elaborate high-tech interventions. Amidst all the cacophony, we seldom hear that there might come a time, later in life, to stop screening for particular diseases. Rarely do we learn that as we age, a different set of conditions, not those customarily tested for, pose a major threat to well-being.

What is newsworthy, by contrast, is the widespread inadequacy of access to medical care—45 million Americans are uninsured, patients living in rural areas may be two hours away from sophisticated treatment, black patients are less likely than whites to undergo bypass surgery—a reality so disturbing that it overshadows another alarming truth: at the same time that we fail to provide the most rudimentary care to some, we lavish unnecessary medical care on others.[2] But if the baby boomers are to have a good old age, we will need to stop squandering resources on tests and treatments that offer little or no benefit—and sometimes cause considerable pain and suffering—and concentrate instead on interventions that can truly improve quality of life.

BARBARA AND LEWIS DELRAY had come to my office to lodge a complaint. Lewis's father, a dapper retired engineer living with his wife in an upscale retirement community, had recently seen his physician for a routine physical examination. He had felt fine; it was simply time, as he put it, for an oil change. And since he had just turned 80, he figured he was due for a bit of routine maintenance, something analogous to the 60,000-mile tune-up his mechanic had just given to his 1990 Buick Regal. His physician was a personable young man, with Ivy League credentials and clothing to match, though perhaps a tad too preppy for his taste. According to Mr. Delray Senior, the entire exam had taken no more than twenty minutes. Moreover, when he received the results of his lab tests in the mail, together with a form letter telling him what a pleasure it had been to meet him, he realized they didn't include a prostate specific antigen (PSA) level. He had always had the prostate cancer test, ever since it had been discovered. And, he noted, his physician had not recommended a colonoscopy, another test he was accustomed to having regularly. On the contrary, the doctor had intimated that the colonoscopy he had had five years earlier would suffice for at least another five years, if not indefinitely.

Mr. Delray reported to his son that he felt short-changed. The new doctor—for he was a recent addition to the staff of the retirement community's health center—was a nice enough fellow, but he was not *thorough*. Barbara and Lewis were outraged.

I was in charge of the medical care at the continuing-care retirement community where Mr. Delray lived. It was a large campus that included apartments for vigorous older people, other apartments for elders needing a little more day-to-day help, and a skilled nursing facility in case the residents needed considerable help. In fact, I had hired the physician in question and had recently introduced him to his prospective patients at an elegant reception attended by various local dignitaries, including the congressman from the district and the CEO of the health care system of which the retirement community was a part. It was my job to explain to the Delrays just what I planned to do to rectify the manifest deficiencies of my staff.

Barbara was wearing an aquamarine wool suit, with color-coordinated leather shoes. Her hair was perfectly coiffed; despite the windy weather, each strand had remained in place. With not a single gray hair and no wrinkles, she looked to be about 40. But when she turned her head and the light struck her face from the side, I noticed that she was heavily made up, and I thought I glimpsed a few pale roots. Barbara, I soon learned, was the executive vice president of a large and successful software firm. She had plenty of money for Botox injections and visits to the beauty parlor to color her hair. I revised my estimate: closer to 60 than to 40.

Lewis exuded lawyerliness with his plain white shirt, dark suit, and shoes that were surely as uncomfortable as they were expensive. The only splash of color was an uncharacteristically flashy Jerry Garcia tie. I later heard that his law firm had represented the "Dead" in a lawsuit, and the band had demonstrated their gratefulness by giving each partner a tie after winning a generous settlement. Lewis was so quiet that he made me nervous—I had no idea what he was thinking. His firm did not handle malpractice cases, and in any event there could be no question of litigation since Mr. Delray had not suffered any harm. A week after his unsatisfactory appointment with the physician in my employ, he was seen in a nearby private medical office. In that establishment, as he put it, he had every one of his orifices examined. He also underwent a comprehensive battery of screening tests, including a PSA.

The problem was, Barbara continued, that his PSA had been elevated. The normal range is up to 4, with levels of 4 to 10 moderately concerning and levels over 10 often, though not invariably, associated with cancer. Mr. Delray's level had been 12.

I told Barbara and Lewis that I regretted Mr. Delray Senior had been dissatisfied with his experience, and that I would transmit their concerns to the physician in question. But I also commented that screening for prostate cancer with a PSA test was not generally recommended for 80-year-olds. In fact, most of the existing guidelines did not recommend it for men over 70 and some, such as the Canadian guidelines, did not suggest it for anyone.[3] Too often, the test leads to a false-positive result: the PSA is elevated but the patient does not have cancer. Even more disturbing is the fact that many people who do turn out to have prostate cancer, and then undergo aggressive curative therapy, die of heart problems or kidney problems or some other malignancy well before the prostate has time to produce symptoms.

Barbara Delray made it very clear that she was not interested in statistics. She did not care what was right *in general.* Her father-in-law was not a data point. He had been at risk of developing cancer. He had gotten cancer. He was going to have it treated. And if he had gone along with my staff doctor's recommendations, he would never even have been diagnosed.

Barbara wanted the doctor fired. Lewis explained calmly that they both cared deeply about the retirement community. Though their family member had survived despite his completely inadequate physical examination, they wanted to save the other residents of the community, who were perhaps less savvy than Elliott Delray, from gross incompetence. I indicated that I would perform a full review of the new doctor's performance, taking into consideration feedback from patients and families as well as an objective review of his medical records. I thanked them for their concern, reiterated how pleased I was that Mr. Delray had found another physician more to his liking, and escorted the indignant duo out of my office.

SINCE THE 1920s, the American medical establishment has extolled the virtues of the annual checkup. The American Medical

Association first proposed a comprehensive annual physical examination for all adults, including diagnostic tests, in 1922.[4] Not until the 1970s was the wisdom of this approach challenged, when a handful of physicians asked the radical question: What is the evidence that annual exams accomplish what they are supposed to? After poring through the medical literature, the Canadian Task Force on the Periodic Health Examination observed that only a small number of preventive health care interventions have been scientifically shown to be sound. These tests, the Task Force argued, could be done during sick visits and did not justify an annual physical examination.[5] Within a few years, the American College of Physicians, the United States Preventive Services Task Force, and even the American Medical Association came around to the view that regular checkups should be abandoned in favor of a more selective way of preventing disease.

Members of today's older generation have heard about the alleged benefits of a "complete" examination for fifty years. Not surprisingly, it is what they expect from their physicians. In fact, a recent study of residents of three American cities, Denver, San Diego, and Boston, found that the overwhelming majority of adults thought this kind of complete physical exam constitutes good medical care. A total of 1,203 people answered a telephone questionnaire about their attitudes, with 66 percent asserting unequivocally that an annual examination is essential for staying healthy. They had a clear idea of what that exam should entail: it should include a blood pressure check, a heart and lung exam, an abdominal exam, a prostate exam (for men), and a test of their reflexes. The U.S. Preventive Services Task Force, by contrast, recommends that of these, only the blood pressure be checked yearly. Fully 90 percent of the men responding to the questionnaire wanted a prostate specific antigen test, a blood count, and a test for diabetes, although none of these is recommended on a routine basis.[6]

What I found particularly disturbing about this study was that the few screening tests that have been shown scientifically to make a difference were precisely the tests that the patients surveyed were not especially eager to have. Sigmoidoscopy, which has been convincingly shown to detect colon cancer at a treatable stage, was acceptable to only 30 percent of patients. Pap smears were accepted by 75 percent of women. The acceptance rate for the non-recommended tests was far higher. Just how important —or unimportant—screening tests were to most patients was driven home by the finding that as soon as a charge was imposed for the test, the patients lost interest in having it done. If patients had to pay $150 for an annual exam, for instance, suddenly the percentage of people who wanted one dropped to 33 percent. The interest in Pap smears and mammograms fell about 50 percent if there was a fee. The public view of what constitutes good medical care and the opinion of professional medical societies appear to diverge considerably.

Regular visits to physicians do play an important role in good medical care, but not because doctors perform a detailed physical exam. The primary reason the annual visit is important is that it allows the physician and patient to get to know each other and to establish a trusting relationship so that the physician will be in a better position to help if and when illness develops. Those screening tests that make sense from a scientific point of view are more likely to get done if the patient is not acutely ill at the time of the visit. And a variety of screening tests that older patients do not currently expect but that may be of great value to them, such as hearing tests and memory evaluations, can be done easily. Routine physical examinations indirectly promote more healthful behavior, but not because physicians regularly uncover unsuspected and treatable problems by listening to lungs and checking reflexes. As an editorial in the *Annals of Internal Medicine,* the journal that published the survey of patient expectations, put it: "If careful study documents that patients who get annual examinations feel better, behave healthier, undergo more appropriate screening, and trust their physicians more than patients who do not have annual examinations, skeptics would need to reconsider the value of this yearly ritual."[7]

What I am saying, as I tried to convey to the Delrays, is that the ingredients of routine health care should be determined by what matters for health. This approach is what is known as "evidence-based medicine." Relying on evidence-based medicine means demanding a scientific basis for deciding whether and in whom a test or treatment is useful. The alternative—deciding what to do on the basis of intuition and common sense—leads to harmful mistakes when it comes to diagnosing and treating disease. The proliferation of screening tests as we age will not result in better health, and may even result in worse health since these tests may lead to additional invasive tests and treatments that come with a host of noxious side effects. Adding ever more tests to the menu of a routine exam will also, in the aggregate, be extremely expensive. If the baby boomers are to have a good old age, then the attitudes and expectations of both patients and physicians toward routine health maintenance (annual physical exams, screening tests, and preventive medicine) need to change radically. We need to adopt a new perspective on routine health care that focuses on targeted screening (for those conditions in which screening has clear benefit), that places value on maintaining quality of life, and that fosters strong relationships between patients and their physicians.

The importance of using evidence-based medicine became apparent as soon as tried-and-true remedies were subjected to careful study. Physicians quickly discovered that many standard approaches were actually no better than a placebo. Anecdotal observations and common sense are just not up to the task of evaluating the efficacy of medical treatment. Because of the inadequacy of mere intuition, new treatments are increasingly tested by means of a randomized double-blind study. In this approach, comparable individuals with the same disorder—ideally of the same severity—are randomly chosen to receive the treatment under study or a control treatment (a sugar pill, in the case of medication). Only if the patients treated with the active chemical do better than the others is the treatment considered effective—and "doing better" means doing measurably better, where "better" is rigorously defined using statistical methods.[8]

Orthopedic surgery, for example, was widely used for the treatment of arthritis of the knee on the basis of common sense rather than science. Osteoarthritis, or wear-and-tear arthritis, is a tremendously common condition, afflicting principally people over the age of 65. Its most debilitating symptom is pain, though when it is very severe, it can also cause difficulty in walking. The standard approach to treatment of osteoarthritis is to start with medication for the pain, such as acetaminophen or anti-inflammatory medicines. If mild medication does not work, the next step is stronger analgesics. Ice, exercise, and injections are also used to try to ameliorate the pain of osteoarthritis. When none of these modalities succeed, physicians search for a more radical means of helping their patients. Some orthopedists hit upon the plausible idea that if they mechanically cleaned out the joint, patients would feel considerably better. Because it seemed so sensible, the procedure known as "lavage and debridement"—literally cleaning and scraping, carried out through a small instrument known as an arthroscope—was readily adopted. After the anesthesiologist puts the patient to sleep, the orthopedist makes a small incision into the knee joint, inserting a special instrument that enables him to see into the joint. He then scrapes the surface of the joint and flushes out any debris.

By the year 2000, more than 650,000 of these procedures were being performed each year, at a cost of about $5000 per procedure. Then, for the first time, a few courageous physicians decided to formally study the procedure by randomly assigning patients to receive arthroscopy with lavage, arthroscopy with debridement, or sham surgery. The doctors did not tell patients which procedure had been done, nor did they notify the physicians who assessed the outcomes. The researchers evaluated both groups with objective tests of pain and of walking and stair climbing. Astonishingly, after following the 165 patients who completed the trial for two years, the investigators found no difference between the groups in either their reports of pain or their ability to walk.[9] Although various technical objections to the study were raised, they were fairly minor and hardly compelling enough to justify putting hundreds of thousands of patients through surgery at a cost of $3.25 billion yearly.[10] A number of commentators raised questions about the ethics of doing sham surgery, even though all the patients were informed that they would either receive the real thing or simulated surgery, and the subjects all agreed to participate. The investigators and the editors of the *New England Journal of Medicine* defended their respective decisions to perform and publish the study on the grounds that common sense had suggested the procedure was effective, and only a controlled test could answer the question of whether common sense was correct.

Perhaps where the physician went wrong with Mr. Delray was that he did not explain *why* he performed only a limited physical examination or *why* he only ordered certain screening tests. But it is likely that Mr. Delray would have been skeptical about his doctor's motivation, wondering perhaps whether he was trying to save money for Medicare. Or, more fundamentally, he might have been suspicious of science itself. After all, how can physicians legitimately claim to provide care based on the latest data when the data change all the time? In some years cholesterol is bad for you, and in other years only certain kinds of cholesterol are bad. During my second pregnancy, I wasn't supposed to drink coffee because it could harm my baby, whereas previously, when I was pregnant with my first child, and subsequently, when I was carrying my third, I could drink as much coffee as I liked.

The estrogen story is even more dramatic. For many years,

estrogen was considered a wonder drug for post-menopausal women. It effectively combated debilitating and unpleasant hot flashes, its initial purpose, while simultaneously preventing osteoporosis, heart disease, and dementia. The only adverse consequence of taking estrogen appeared to be an increased risk of developing uterine cancer. That potential problem was irrelevant to women who had had a hysterectomy, and could readily be surmounted by combining estrogen with another hormone, progesterone, in women who had not.

But in 1998, results from the first randomized study of estrogen use began to emerge, and they indicated that estrogen did not prevent heart attacks. On the contrary, it increased the risk of assorted medical problems including blood clots in the veins (deep vein thrombosis) and the lungs (pulmonary embolism). The next large study to come along, the Women's Health Initiative, showed that not only did estrogen fail to prevent heart attacks, but it seemed to *cause* heart attacks, as well as strokes, pulmonary emboli, and breast cancer. The news went from bad to worse, and by 2002, the *Annals of Internal Medicine* ran an editorial with the title: "Post-Menopausal Hormone Replacement Therapy: How Could We Have Been So Wrong?"[11] How indeed could this have happened?

For years, the only information about estrogen came from observational studies, studies in which some women chose, for reasons of their own, to use estrogen, and others chose not to. Women were not randomly assigned to take estrogen or a placebo. Researchers monitored outcomes: they looked at whether women were more likely to develop heart attacks or hip fractures in one group than in the other. Since the women in the two groups might be different in important ways that could influence the results, statisticians attempted to compensate for the differences in age, race, and diet. The problem with this kind of adjustment is that it requires making all sorts of assumptions about just how much those differences matter. The second problem is that we do not always know what factors to adjust for. Suppose that age at first pregnancy turns out to affect the risk of getting breast cancer (it does), but suppose we didn't know that. If the group of estrogen-takers happened to include a great many women who had children at a young age, it would look as though estrogen use lowered the risk of breast cancer when in fact it was the age of their first pregnancy that mattered. Only when a large study was carried out consisting of women who were randomized to take estrogen or a placebo did the finding emerge that estrogen did not do many of the things we thought it did. As a result, a rational choice about estrogen use in 2005 is not the same as a rational choice was in 1995. The conclusion is not that women should decide whether to take estrogen depending on their gut feeling; rather, the conclusion is that the right decision depends on having the most up-to-date information.

Evidence-based medicine is necessary because medicine is too complex and the number of possible treatments too vast for clinicians and patients to rely solely on their own judgment. The challenge, with respect to periodic physical examinations, is to apply evidence-based medicine to the particular patient. Barbara Delray wanted to make sure that physicians treated her father-in-law as a unique individual, that he wasn't just "a number." The way to do that is not to throw out science and substitute intuition; instead, it is to incorporate values and preferences as well as data into decision making.

The saga of Elliott Delray did not come to an end when his son and daughter-in-law marched out of my office, incensed that he had not been given a complete physical examination and determined to see justice done. I continued to hear from Lewis about each new development as it occurred. In what was a remarkable infringement of confidentiality, Lewis sent monthly bulletins updating me on his father's medical condition. First I received a pathology report: six biopsy samples had been taken in the urologist's office, using an ultrasound machine to locate the irregular areas on the surface of the gland that were most suspicious for tumor. Of the six pieces of tissue, four showed cancer. Based on the microscopic analysis of the tissue, Mr. Delray had a reasonably good prognosis. Next I saw abdominal CAT scan reports and bone scan results, which showed that the cancer did not appear to have spread beyond the prostate. Then I received a discharge summary from Mr. Delray's hospitalization for a radical prostatectomy. A "post-it" note was attached, on which Lewis had scribbled, "He's cured!"

The correspondence from the Delrays stopped at that point, but I continued to receive information from other sources. I next got a concerned call from the manager of the continuing-care retirement community: Mr. Delray was now incontinent. The other residents did not want him coming to the dining room anymore because he dribbled. He smelled. The chairs on which he had sat smelled. The director of housekeeping was in despair: Mr. Delray's apartment reeked of urine. The staff knew the Delrays were angry at the facility and did not want to alienate them further by suggesting that Mr. Delray have his incontinence evaluated, or that he move out of his apartment in the independent living section and into the assisted living unit.

Putting the memo on top of my stack of fairly urgent "to do" items, I set off to attend our weekly medical conference where we discuss challenging medical cases. On the agenda was a psychiatric case, and I looked forward to the diversion from internal medicine. My psychiatric colleague reported he had been treating a charming 78-year-old woman for depression, hardly an uncommon problem in older people. But the reason he wanted to discuss the case, the reason he found it both poignant and enlightening, is that his patient had revealed during a recent therapy session that her depressive symptoms began when her husband was diagnosed with prostate cancer. Her husband wasn't depressed, as we might have expected. She wasn't worried that her husband might die, a potential explanation for depression. She was confident the disease had been caught early, in plenty of time. Her husband had had the best, most definitive treatment. But since his surgery, he had been impotent. Elliott wasn't a dirty old man, Mrs. Delray said defensively. They simply enjoyed their sex life together. They always had. And overnight, it had been destroyed.

With the newest "nerve-sparing" techniques used in radical prostatectomy, incontinence and impotence are not as common as they are with conventional surgery, but they remain frequent complications.[12] When radiation treatment is used to treat prostate cancer, an approach associated with a decreased chance of developing incontinence, intractable diarrhea may ensue instead. Because the side effects accompanying definitive treatment are noxious, and because many men with prostate cancer never develop widespread disease and many others go on for years before the disease progresses, some men choose to adopt a course of "watchful waiting." They only accept treatment if the PSA begins to climb further or if they develop new symptoms. Many men do not have their PSA measured in the first place, particularly those with a life expectancy of less than ten years.[13]

Mr. Delray made an appointment to see his urologist about his incontinence. Maybe if he felt bold, he would mention the impotence. The appointment wasn't scheduled for another six weeks— his urologist was a busy man, and the mildly unpleasant side effects of a life-saving procedure hardly constituted an emergency. In the meantime, his friends and neighbors avoided him. He spent more and more time in his apartment, though he grudgingly wore an adult diaper to catch any leaks. His wife confessed to the psychiatrist that she had been tempted to put her antidepressant pills in his coffee.

Elliott Delray never saw the urologist. He died of a massive heart attack before the scheduled appointment. I read his obituary in the newspaper.

SCREENING tests, like the comprehensive physical examination, should be subjected to scientific scrutiny. The logic of screening rests on the assumption that finding something early is always a good thing. Thus, screening tests such as mammograms or the prostate specific antigen are widely assumed to be beneficial. The reality, however, is that "catching it early" is not always useful. It is only helpful if there is an effective treatment for the disease that is "caught." Otherwise, "catching it early" means knowing for a longer period that you have an incurable disease. And if there is a cure, you should make sure that you don't have some other condition that is likely to get to you long before the "curable" disease does. The mania for early diagnosis is dramatically illustrated by one of the newest screening tests on the market, the total body scan.

Driving home recently, I heard an advertisement on the radio for the "Be-Well Body Scan." This turns out to be a local brand name for a three-dimensional X-ray that promises to pinpoint heart disease and cancers at a very early stage. The body scan lets physicians look inside the human body with greater precision than ever before. Each organ can be scrutinized for aberrant growth, each major blood vessel for possibly dangerous narrowing. The conventional approach to diagnosing and treating disease, by contrast, is either to await the development of symptoms (at which point the disease may be too advanced to be curable) or to try to detect disease by hunting for clues (measuring levels of chemicals that a tumor produces or looking for blood in the stool).

The scanning technique seems patently superior to its predecessors. The X-rays developed by Roentgen in 1905, which today are referred to as "plain films," give only a hazy, two-dimensional view of the body's mysteries. More recent radiological techniques such as computerized axial tomography (CAT) scans and ultrasound tests permit physicians to home in on whatever body parts they wish to examine—the gallbladder or the kidney or the leg veins—if symptoms point in a particular direction. But until the body scan, no single other test gave a detailed view of the entire body. In theory, the scan enables physicians to do during life what the autopsy lets them do after death. The assumption is that hidden within the previously impenetrable body are all kinds of secrets, and that revealing those secrets will be in the best interest of the patient.

The advertisement I heard exhorted healthy people to schedule a scan. I wondered why I didn't know anything about this test, and why it is not covered by health insurance and does not require a physician referral. A little research told me why: there is no scientific evidence that the abnormalities that are detected by such scans are true abnormalities or, if they are real, that the people whose bodies harbor them will live longer or better if the "problems" are excised. As the chairman of radiology at the Massachusetts General Hospital, a major Boston teaching hospital, put it: "It's remarkable to me [that] without any scientific validation whatsoever people are walking in and paying $1000 for this test, which does not even diagnose three of the top four cancers that people get . . . We're waiting for scientific data before marketing these services."[14]

Body scanners have caught on in southern California, perhaps reflecting Hollywood's view of the world as a place where perfect health is achievable. Reportedly, the rich and famous are flocking to be scanned. The body scanner's best publicist is Oprah Winfrey, who labeled it "miraculous" after it detected a plaque in one of her coronary arteries, and who happily displayed her internal organs on the television screen.[15]

If even 10 percent of people aged 65 and older go for a total body scan, the annual cost of the test alone will be over $3 billion, not to mention the cost of training the technicians who do the scans and the radiologists who read them. But the main reason for recommending against screening is not cost. Nor is it failure to detect abnormalities: almost every scan would uncover some kind of abnormality. As one of the first radiologists to advocate widespread use of the total body scan said: "There is not a single human being that I've examined [in whom] I haven't found some evolving pathology."[16] But how would we know whether a kidney lesion was a benign cyst or a malignant tumor? How would we know whether the plaque lining the coronary arteries means an impending heart attack? The only way to know would be to conduct more tests. But we should not recommend those additional tests unless we have evidence that the outcomes with the tests are superior to the outcomes without them.

Elliott Delray, for instance, died of a heart attack long before he had any symptoms from prostate cancer, which often takes ten years to cause problems. The only symptoms he developed were from the *treatment* of his cancer. If the treatment had been devoid of side effects—and there are a few treatments that come with only mild potential side effects—then diagnosis and treatment on the off-chance that it would help might have made sense. But the treatment caused impotence and incontinence. It did not alleviate any other symptoms, and it did not prolong his life.

The principal difficulty with trying to use evidence-based medicine to figure out what screening tests to use in the elderly is the

paucity of relevant data. The scientific data that I have been saying is so very important as the basis for decisions about what tests
to do is minimal for the elderly. The largest, most influential
study of screening for breast cancer, for example, included no
women over the age of 64. Guidelines recently published for
colonoscopy were based on carefully conducted studies of the
outcomes of testing—studies that included people who were
from 50 to 70 years of age.[17]

Medicine has a long history of refusing to extrapolate from
younger people to older ones, only to discover that the benefits
that are well-established in the middle-aged are magnified in
septuagenarians. Treatment of high blood pressure is a case in
point. For years, physicians were reluctant to believe that the
overwhelming benefit of treating high blood pressure that had
been established in the under 65-year-old set was equally applica-
ble to those receiving Medicare. Multiple large epidemiological
trials demonstrated that judicious use of antihypertensive medication markedly reduced the rate of stroke and cardiovascular
death.[18] But doctors came up with all kinds of reasons for believing that the same drugs would not work in older people or would
even be harmful. Atherosclerosis, some argued, turned arteries
into rigid pipes. In order to pump blood through such hard, in-
flexible tubes, high pressures were necessary. Lowering the pressure, or so the argument went, would mean that blood would not
reach the brain, resulting in a stroke—not from excessively high
pressure, but rather from pressure that was effectively too low.
Physicians claimed that their older patients would not be able
to tolerate blood-pressure-lowering medication—drugs that produced a nice, even blood-pressure-lowering effect in younger

people would cause a precipitous drop in pressure when older people stood up, causing them to faint or fall, possibly even breaking a hip in the process.

When a study of blood pressure treatment was finally carried out in people above the age of 65, it showed that the medicines that worked in younger people worked just as well in older ones. In fact, the results were *more* dramatic. These findings have now been confirmed in multiple other trials.[19] Gradually, the medical profession came around to agreeing that vigorous treatment of high blood pressure in older people makes sense.

Just because treating high blood pressure is effective in both old and young people, we can't conclude that *every* treatment and test of proven efficacy in one group will work in the other. The challenge is to figure out when and how to extrapolate from the population in whom a study was done to the specific person we would like to test or treat. The way to face this challenge is to ask, first of all, if there is any physiological reason why what is true for a 50-year-old might not be true for a 75-year-old. Some diseases behave differently at various points during the life cycle or have different epidemiological characteristics. Cervical cancer, for instance, is rare in women over 70. It is almost unheard-of in women over 70 who have had several sequential negative Pap smear tests. Hence, it would not make sense to extrapolate from younger women to older women when screening for cervical cancer. Heart disease, on the other hand, is increasingly common with advancing age. If treating high cholesterol is successful in preventing heart disease in younger people, it is at least plausible to believe it might be effective in an older population.

Patients and families often balk at applying epidemiological data to an individual person. Perhaps if the tests or the therapies were harmless, or better yet cheap and harmless, it might make sense to try anyway, even if the data did not support the intervention. But most tests are not harmless, nor are they cheap—or the screening test may be innocuous, but a positive test is apt to lead to other tests that are both invasive and expensive. Positive mammograms trigger breast biopsies; positive total body scans may precipitate cardiac catheterizations or surgery. We need to start with the science, modulating our approach in accordance with the particular situation of the individual patient, so as not to inflict harm on the individual and the larger society.

The way to go about this is with a highly individualized decision-making strategy. Using this model, when a patient like Elliott Delray shows up in the office for a routine physical exam, I might start by assessing his underlying health status. Far more important than chronological age is the totality of medical conditions that influence a patient's chance of getting through an acute illness, and of living long enough to benefit from screening tests. Mr. Delray, for instance, was in reasonably good shape for an 80-year-old. There was no reason to believe he was dying, and his mind worked perfectly. But he did have a history of high blood pressure, and he had had a heart attack several years earlier; he had diabetes, for which he was taking a pill every day; and he had a history of cigarette smoking, though he had kicked the habit when he moved into the continuing-care retirement community. To judge from his various medical problems, he was probably much like the average 80-year-old man—better off than some, a little sicker than others. The life expectancy of an 80-year-old white man today is typically seven years.[20] What I would say to him is that he was in luck: he didn't need to bother with PSA tests anymore. He had been monitored over the years and had shown no signs of trouble. Prostate cancer typically takes years to progress sufficiently to produce problems. So if he had been fine over the preceding five years, he would probably remain fine, at least in terms of his prostate, for the rest of his life.

On the other hand, if Elliott Delray were 70 years old and in excellent health, I would use a different tack. I would begin by saying that many men were being screened for prostate cancer but there was no strong evidence that this was a good idea. In fact, not a single study had shown that screening could prolong life. Lots of men who have a positive test go on to have a biopsy. Many of the biopsies don't show any evidence of cancer. Some men do have cancerous cells found on biopsy, and many of them then have surgery or radiation, both of which have a fair number of side effects. It wasn't clear, on balance, whether treatment was preferable to a "wait and see" approach. So, I would say, whether you want to be tested depends on how important it is to you to know what's going on, and whether you would want active treatment if we found a tumor.

If Elliott Delray were 70 but had another life-threatening disease, such as moderately severe emphysema or fairly advanced Parkinson's disease, I would take yet another approach. I might say something like: Some men your age get a blood test to check for prostate cancer. We don't have reason to believe this is an effective strategy. I think we should focus on dealing with your other medical problems and not worry about your prostate. If you feel very strongly that you want the test done—perhaps you would find a negative test tremendously reassuring—I can order it for you, but I can't say I recommend it.[21]

Prevention does matter as we age. But just what we are seeking to prevent has to change over time. Currently, we are spending our energy and our resources vainly trying to stave off the wrong conditions. What we should be trying to prevent are things like falls and social isolation, both of which can have extraordinary consequences for older people.

Consider falls among the elderly. "Falling" is not a disease the way breast cancer and pneumonia and multiple sclerosis are diseases. It is not caused by a bacterium or a virus. In fact, it is not "caused" by any single factor. It has the dubious privilege of being a "geriatric syndrome," which is to say it isn't really a single condition at all, but rather any of a number of states, the result of which is a repeated tendency to hit the floor. And falling cannot be attributed to a well-defined cause; instead, it is "multifactorial." Falls occur when the right combination of conditions arise simultaneously to produce the wrong outcome—a little visual impairment comes together with a touch of arthritis in a person taking antidepressant medication, and the result is a nasty tumble down the stairs.

Unlike a toddler's falls, an older person's falls are apt to cause injury. More than a third of people over the age of 65 fall each year, and 10 percent of those who fall sustain a serious injury such as a hip fracture or bleeding into the brain. Even when a fall does not result in physical harm, the faller is often so traumatized, so fearful of falling again, that he stops going out on his own or refuses to leave his home. And when injury does occur, it is often devastating. A broken hip often spells the beginning of the end: of the 350,000 Americans who break a hip every year, only 50 to 65 percent will walk as well as they did before the fall. About 20 percent will never walk again. And if that's not bad enough, nearly 40 percent end up in a nursing home, and 37 percent are dead within a year.[22]

What most people fail to realize is that we can do a great deal to prevent falls. We can't eliminate them altogether, but it turns out that there are risk factors for falling just as there are risk factors for heart disease. In one study, just three factors predicted falls remarkably well: muscle weakness, poor balance, and taking more than four prescription medications. Older people with none of these risk factors had a 12 percent chance of falling in a year, but those with all three were virtually certain to fall.[23]

Physicians can intervene to affect these risk factors. Exercise programs, particularly tai chi, can improve balance and prevent falls. A careful medication review can have powerful consequences: while many drugs have been implicated in falls, the leading offenders are psychiatric medicines, particularly pills to counteract depression and anxiety.[24]

In addition to risk factor modification, which has a modest effect in reducing falls, we can try to decrease the damage that occurs if an elderly person does fall. We can strengthen the bones—by age 70, one-third of women have osteoporosis, or decreased bone mass, which predisposes to fractures, and by age 80, 70 percent of women have osteoporosis.[25] We have medication that can significantly improve bone mass, which translates into a large decrease in fracture rate. And finally, we can recommend hip protectors to the frailest individuals in order to cushion the hip at the time of a fall. With a new, streamlined design and space-age materials, these pads are scarcely noticeable, and they have been shown to cut the fracture rate in half.[26]

Focusing on falls is just one of the many forms of preventive medicine that are underutilized in caring for older people today. Combating social isolation is another fruitful activity, one in which physicians can play an important role, much as they do in helping patients to stop smoking or persuading them to wear seatbelts. The degree of social support and social engagement has a potent effect on a whole host of illnesses, from heart attacks to strokes to hip fractures.[27] Older people are less apt to become disabled and actually less likely to die after hospitalization for any one of these problems if they have regular, meaningful social contacts.[28] And while the mantra "use it or lose it" is too simplistic as an explanation of the cause of dementia, older people who remain engaged with their community are less likely to develop cognitive impairment that those who do not.[29]

The goal of screening tests and physical examinations in old age is not to stave off death, a hopeless and counterproductive aim. In some instances, the goal is not even to prevent disease. Rather, the true goal of medical care in old age is to maintain normal function as long as possible and to postpone the development of disability. Physicians should work with patients to achieve these goals. But we will all need to abandon our anachronistic views of "health maintenance" and agree on preventive strategies tailored to the realities of aging.

TWO

When Less Is More

PREVENTION takes on a new meaning in old age, even for vigorous elders who can look forward to many years of active life. Good prevention means screening for conditions that are seldom found in younger patients, such as cognitive impairment, hearing loss, or falls. And it means ceasing to screen for other disorders that are of little relevance to older people, not out of misguided ageism, but because early detection no longer carries with it a clear benefit and may instead lead to treatment that produces painful or unpleasant symptoms. Just as overtreatment of older individuals is widespread in the sphere of prevention, so too is it a problem in the realm of diagnosing and treating disease. Nowhere are the perils of overtreatment more evident than in caring for the frail elderly.[1]

ONE OF my nursing home patients was in the emergency room. The covering doctor had sent her to the hospital because she had nausea, vomiting, and an anxious daughter. Her daughter hastened to inform my associate that the last time her mother had had an episode of nausea and vomiting, she had been having a heart attack.

I found Mildred Steiner shivering under a sheet and what passed for a blanket. She was lying on a gurney that was covered by a one-inch foam mattress, tucked into a relatively quiet, which is to say moderately hectic, corner of the emergency room. Mildred was blind, slightly demented, and single-minded in her wish to be left alone.

"How are you feeling?" I asked.

"Cold," she told me.

I tried to listen to her heart and lungs but she pushed me away. "Don't you have anything better to do?" she asked. I told her that I was her doctor and that I wanted to help. "You could get me a blanket," she suggested.

Finding a blanket was not trivial, but I finally located a nurse who remembered seeing one mixed in with the sheets. She triumphantly produced a threadbare cotton cover, which I dutifully brought to Mildred. "Thank you, dear," she said. "Now you can go."

I persevered with my questioning but despaired of doing a physical examination now that Mildred had all but disappeared under the newly procured blanket. "Do you have any pain in your chest?"

"I'm fine, dear." She was polite but stubborn.

"Are you still nauseated?"

"There's nothing wrong with me."

I gave up. Casual observation confirmed that she could lie flat without any difficulty breathing—the emergency room pillow was almost as thin as the blanket—a good sign, since heart attacks are often accompanied by fluid in the lungs. I watched the monitor which displayed Mildred's electrocardiogram (EKG) and vital signs. Her heart rate was regular and neither too fast nor too slow, another good sign. A cuff around her thin, flabby arm automatically inflated and deflated every few minutes, revealing that her blood pressure was a healthy 130/60. And the squiggly line denoting her cardiac rhythm looked remarkably normal. Appearances can be deceiving, but Mildred Steiner did not look like someone in the throes of a heart attack.

Conceivably she could have had a heart attack earlier, back at the nursing home. I logged onto the hospital computer to see if any laboratory test results were ready. There was one: a urinalysis. Her urine was loaded with white blood cells and bacteria, strongly suggesting a urinary tract infection, which often produces nausea.

Armed with this information, I tracked down the emergency room physician and suggested that we obtain a single blood test, a CPK-MB band, which is characteristically elevated when a person is having an acute myocardial infarction. Since Mildred did not appear clinically to be having a heart attack, and since the abnormal urinalysis provided a plausible explanation for her symptoms, I reasoned that a normal blood test would provide a little more confirmatory evidence. If the CPK turned out to be elevated, we would admit Mildred to the hospital and "rule out" a myocardial infarction: she would have serial blood tests and EKGs. She would be hooked up to a cardiac monitor on a unit with experienced nurses and specialized equipment to deal with heart attacks and their complications. If the CPK was negative, we would send her back to the nursing home and treat her with oral antibiotics for a urinary tract infection.

"You can't just order one CPK," I was told. "You have to order three, spread out over 24 hours." It is true that the *usual* protocol is to obtain three sequential blood tests. The CPK-MB level, while highly sensitive for cardiac damage, may take 3 to 4 hours to become elevated. A normal test could be misleading.[2] For most patients, if there is sufficient concern about a possible heart attack, the best approach is to hospitalize them, attach them to a cardiac monitor to watch for irregular heart rhythms, and test their blood the mandated three times. But what if the patient is a confused older woman from a nursing home who turns out to have a fever and a urinary tract infection, which can readily be treated at the nursing home? The chance that she has had a heart attack *in addition* is small. Moreover, the price of admitting her to the hospital just to be sure is that she will become more confused and very frightened. If a single negative blood test would lower the possibility that she had had a heart attack even further—from 20 percent to 10 percent, say—given that we already had an explanation for her malaise and given that her electrocardiogram was unchanged from the one done a month earlier, wasn't that a reasonable strategy?

I had no choice. I admitted Mildred to the hospital. I knew she would be subject to all the adverse effects of hospitalization in people who are frail: confusion and a cascade of complications resulting in increased disability. I knew those risks could be moderated only slightly by good geriatric care. A geriatric approach strives to prevent acute confusion (delirium) by avoiding delirium-inducing medication; it attempts to counteract disability by prescribing vigorous in-hospital exercises; and it seeks to avoid physician-induced complications (iatrogenesis) by thorough and assiduous attention to detail. These efforts can probably reduce the chance that hospitalization will result in a bad outcome, but to date such reductions have been modest. An admirable, multi-component strategy to decrease the incidence of delirium in hospitalized elderly patients managed to lower the rate only from 15 to 10 percent. Likewise, strategies aimed at mobilizing inpatients early rather than accepting the inevitable deconditioning that arises from prolonged bed rest have led to slight decreases in the percentage of elders requiring permanent nursing home care.[3] Such attempts at palliation, while clearly better than nothing for hospitalized patients, do not do away with the adverse effects of hospital care.

The more radical approach would be to avoid hospitalization altogether. Rather than proceed with "usual care" while trying to minimize its deleterious consequences, why not simply avoid "usual care"? If hospitals are toxic to older people, why not try to treat them at home rather than administer antitoxins? If the benefit of the hospital—the presence of physicians and nurses 24 hours a day and of monitoring equipment—is also the source of the toxicity, then attempts at detoxification are destined to fail.

Just as there is a gap between the scientific view of routine health maintenance and the popular view, so too there is a gap between the geriatric approach to health care for the frail older adult and the general view. The conventional wisdom is that patients should receive the treatment most likely to extend life, no matter how unpleasant or debilitating the side effects—or else forgo treatment altogether and opt for hospice care. This view is very simple, black and white with no gray. In actuality, there is a middle ground between maximally aggressive care and exclusively comfort-oriented care, and many frail elders would benefit from precisely this brand of *intermediate* care. If we are to experience a good old age, we will need a broader range of options than those that currently prevail.

The belief that there is only one right approach to treatment of acute illness is pervasive. I have talked to surgeons who are convinced that the correct treatment for an acute gallbladder attack (cholecystitis) is surgery, and anything short of surgery is almost unthinkable. And in fact the standard, approved treatment for cholecystitis is intravenous antibiotics followed by an operation to remove the gallbladder. The reason for this approach is that many patients will relapse if they do not have the gallbladder taken out—they have a 70 percent chance of recurrence of symptoms over the next two years.[4] Given this high risk, it appears logical to proceed immediately with surgery, particularly if the patient is otherwise healthy. But what about an 80-year-old patient with cholecystitis? Should she go ahead with surgery if she has multiple other medical problems, which make her a poor surgical candidate? Should she proceed, even though she might have a protracted period of recuperation, spending three weeks of the few years of active life she has left in a skilled nursing facility and then another three—or four or five—months convalescing at home? Or should she take her chances with intravenous antibiotics alone? What if she, like Mildred Steiner, already lived in a nursing home and just wanted to be left alone? I have treated a number of very frail older people with this condition conservatively, using antibiotics for the acute gallbladder inflammation and then following an approach of watchful waiting. Many of those patients died of something else, sometimes a year or two later, before their gallbladders ever acted up again.

The medical profession tends not to consider intermediate care because physicians assume that patients are interested either in life-prolongation or in comfort care. Even the Study to Understand Prognoses and Preferences for Care (SUPPORT), an influential, widely cited study of preferences for care in seriously ill hospitalized adults, offered patients only two choices, curative care or comfort care.[5] What is not acknowledged is that there may be several ways to seek to extend life, perhaps not of equal efficacy but each with a discrete set of side effects. Some side effects may be so undesirable that a patient would prefer the somewhat less effective treatment rather than risk the adverse effect associated with the slightly more effective treatment.

Preferences regarding side effects clearly matter if there is a choice between two treatments that are, on average, equally effective. Treatment of cancer of the larynx, for example, involves either removal of the larynx or radiation treatment. Surgery eliminates the ability to speak and exposes the patient to the risk of death in the short run (as a result of operative complications). Radiotherapy preserves speech and is not associated with short-term complications, but in the long term it is associated with a shorter survival. Depending on their preference, some patients might gamble that they will come through the surgery and adapt to an artificial voice box; others might choose to risk a shorter life but not incur the chance of immediate death or loss of speech.[6]

Preferences also clearly matter if the side effects are sufficiently severe. When asked whether they would want a life-prolonging treatment if the cost were dementia, four out of five in one group of elderly New Haven residents said they were uninterested. Similarly, if the price for life-prolongation was total dependence on other people, nearly three-quarters of the older people interviewed said no to life-prolonging therapy.[7]

Surely preferences also matter if patients have a choice between two treatments with slightly different success rates and markedly different side-effect profiles. I am not talking now about two essentially equivalent treatments—say treatments with only a 5 percent difference in efficacy. Nor am I talking about two treatments with dramatically different outcomes—one that has a 90 percent chance of succeeding and one that has a 10 percent chance. Suppose we can offer two forms of therapy: one approach that has a 60 percent chance of working and another that has a 40 percent chance. In other words, neither is certain to work and neither is certain to fail. The treatment with the 60 percent odds involves hospitalization, surgery, and a prolonged recovery period, whereas the treatment with the 40 percent odds entails intravenous therapy in the nursing home where the patient lives. For many elderly people, the somewhat better odds of the more aggressive strategy would not warrant the acute pain and disorientation, the lengthy recuperation, and the ultimate decline to a lower level of functioning inherent in the more aggressive approach.

"Intermediate care" is not for everyone. Vigorous elders, regardless of age, can expect to fare as well (or as poorly) as their younger counterparts when treated with standard medical care. The benefits may not be quite as great for a person who is 80 as for someone who is 60 simply because the older person has a shorter life expectancy, no matter what treatment is undertaken. But the risks are comparable for robust older people and robust younger people. The many complications of conventional treatment that diminish its appeal to the elderly arise not so much because of age as because of frailty. It is the woman with mild Alzheimer's disease who tends to get confused in the hospital, not the otherwise robust elder with pneumonia. The patient with Alzheimer's disease already has memory problems and disorientation, and these are apt to get worse from fever or pain medication. It is the man with five different chronic diseases and tenuous reserves who becomes debilitated and dependent in the hospital. He is unable to face the stress of an acute gastrointestinal bleed. He goes in with one problem, an ulcer, and develops several more—perhaps a heart attack and congestive heart failure—and emerges too weak to care for himself.

Not all frail older people are interested in intermediate care, even though they are at risk of doing poorly with usual care. Some people may be willing to gamble that they will not be the ones who develop a series of complications, since after all not everybody runs into trouble. Or they may be willing to incur complications, whether a bout of confusion or a heart attack or a hospital-acquired infection, in exchange for the possibility, however small, of living a little longer. They may not view greater dependence, even if it necessitates nursing home care, as sufficiently undesirable to warrant forgoing the most that medical care has to offer.

What I find is that while some frail older people would reject intermediate care as inadequate, most are simply not offered the choice. Their doctors typically give them no alternatives. Starting in the emergency room, while the patient is lying on a stretcher, cold and anxious, the doctor tells him, "you need to come into the hospital," or simply "we're admitting you." The physician then admits the patient and performs a slew of diagnostic tests with the explanation that "we need to do an angiogram" or "we're going to do an endoscopy." The only alternative the hospital physician can imagine is to abandon all potentially curative treatment and focus exclusively on comfort.

If intermediate care is so eminently reasonable, if frail older patients would endorse such an approach in large numbers, why don't their doctors offer it to them? The psychological answer is that physicians are taught to target their efforts to prolonging life—beginning in medical school, where students are told that death is the enemy.[8] And if practicing physicians have any lingering doubts, they are quickly quashed by report cards that rate hospitals on the basis of mortality statistics. Hospitals with higher death rates are classified as inferior to those with lower rates, regardless of whether patients declined potentially life-sustaining interventions.[9] The Medicare program has several times proposed rating individual physicians in the same way and publishing those statistics. The data would be corrected to take into account the age of patients and how sick they were, to try to prevent physicians from being penalized for caring for the sickest, oldest patients, but rarely is it suggested that the data be modified to take patient preferences into account.[10]

Not only are physicians taught that the goal of medicine is to stave off death; they are also instructed that the right way to practice medicine is to begin by clearly and unequivocally establishing a diagnosis and only then considering treatment options. But in the frail older person, the price of obtaining certainty may be exorbitant, as I thought it was for Mildred Steiner. Ideally, we could identify alternative forms of treatment that are just as effective as conventional care without the side effects. A striking example involves alternatives to surgery that are noninvasive or minimally invasive. Most of the complications from a cholecystectomy (surgical removal of the gallbladder), for example, result from the extensive nature of the surgery: the duration of the anesthesia, the size of the abdominal incision, and the length of the recovery period. When the same procedure is done through a laparoscope, the incision is tiny, the hospitalization drops from a week to two days, and the effects on stamina and mobility are markedly decreased. A similar argument can be made for substituting stenting for coronary artery bypass surgery. During placement of a stent, the patient remains awake. The cardiologist administers a local anesthetic at the site where he threads a catheter into a groin artery and from there into the coronary artery. Next, the physician injects dye to locate the narrowed area of the artery, and then inserts a small wire mesh into the blood vessel to hold it open and allow better blood flow. Contrast this procedure with bypass surgery, in which the surgeon cracks open the chest, puts the patient on a heart-bypass machine so that he can empty the heart of blood, and then takes a vein from the leg and sews it between the two healthy parts of the affected coronary artery. Although recovery from open heart surgery is often remarkably quick, perhaps because an incision in the chest causes fewer mobility problems than does an abdominal incision, being "on the pump" may cause cognitive deficits.[11]

For select patients, laparoscopic cholecystectomy and cardiac stents are just as effective as the original procedures, with fewer side effects. And even if the outcome in terms of life-prolongation is not quite as good with these less invasive approaches, patients might be willing to trade off quantity of life for quality.

SAM DRYDEN was my patient in the transitional care unit, also called a subacute unit, a small, ten-bed section of a nursing home where he was recovering from a heart attack. An 88-year-old widower, Sam had gone to his local community hospital after waking up in the middle of the night with chest pain. He had waited an hour, telling himself it was just heartburn, and then another hour, telling himself the pain was getting better and would go away soon. When the pain was as severe as ever after three hours, and Sam was starting to sweat and to feel short of breath, he called an ambulance.

Sam remained in the coronary care unit of the hospital for two days, just long enough for the doctors to conclude that he had had another heart attack (it was his fourth), to put him on blood-thinning medicine to try to prevent a fifth, and to add a new heart medication to his already impressive regimen. As soon as they decided he was stable, the doctors transferred Sam to a regular medical floor. After a day of further testing—he had an echocardiogram to determine how well his heart was pumping and another chest X-ray because the initial film, taken in the emergency room, looked as though a tumor might be lurking in his lung behind his heart—the young intern on the team wanted to send Sam home. Sam was eager to go: he liked his two-bedroom apartment with the black and white television he'd had for twenty years, his collection of jazz records, and his own bed. But when he got up and tried to walk down the corridor for the first time since entering the hospital, he became dizzy. He turned pale and would have fallen if an alert nurse hadn't grabbed him. She paged the intern and told him forcefully that Sam Dryden was in no condition to go home. Just because his repeat chest X-ray was negative and he hadn't had any further chest pain in 24 hours didn't mean he was able to make it on his own. Instead, the hospital referred him to a skilled nursing facility, where he went to regain his strength.

I had only met Sam once when I was called to see him again. "He looks awful," the nurse told me. Anne was a seasoned nurse, an excellent clinician, and a wise person. If she said my patient was in bad shape, I needed to see him urgently. When I arrived on the floor, Sam was ashen. Beads of perspiration dotted his forehead. His breathing was labored. He was sitting bolt upright in bed. He looked as though he had been running away from a mugger and that his assailant was gaining on him.

"Are you having chest pain?" I asked. He nodded. "Trouble breathing?" He nodded again.

"His blood pressure is 80/50," Anne told me quietly. That was much too low. I couldn't safely give him nitroglycerine, which could cause his pressure to drop even further. "Heart rate's 80." His heart rate had been running around 60 as a result of the beta-blocker he was taking, so a rate of 80 meant his heart was racing.

I quickly listened to his lungs: he had evidence of a little fluid buildup, as often happens if the heart isn't pumping well. On examining his heart, I heard an extra sound, a "gallop," also suggestive of a struggling heart. Just as I was about to request that we get an electrocardiogram, the technician walked in, wheeling her EKG machine. I smiled gratefully at Anne, who had anticipated my request. "Respiratory therapy is on the way with oxygen and to check his level," she added, reading my mind again.

The EKG showed ischemia, an acute lack of oxygen to the heart. Coming so quickly on the heels of his recent heart attack, the reading was ominous. "I think you should go to the hospital," I told Sam.

"I don't want to go back to that place I went last time," Sam answered. "I want to go where my cardiologist is." I said I would tell the ambulance driver to take him to the hospital where he usually received his care, but sometimes they had to bring patients to the nearest facility.

"You mean I'm that bad?" he asked.

"They just want to get help for you quickly," I answered lamely.

"I don't want to die," Sam added.

"You're going to be okay." I squeezed his hand. "I expect you back in a couple of days."

When I called the hospital the next day for an update on Sam, I learned he had gone directly from the emergency room to the cardiac catheterization lab. The cardiologists had injected dye into his coronary arteries and discovered that he had multiple blockages. The main artery feeding the left ventricle, the most critical part of his heart, was almost totally obstructed. The recommended treatment was coronary artery bypass surgery, a major procedure for anyone but a particularly daunting prospect for an 88-year-old man with limited kidney and lung function as well. The Dryden family were thinking about whether to authorize surgery, I was told. While they were thinking, the cardiologists placed Sam on intra-aortic balloon pump counterpulsation, a high-tech way of helping his heart to keep on going.

Five days later, Sam Dryden returned to the transitional care unit. He was tired and didn't remember much about his hospital stay. His time in the coronary care unit, attached to the balloon pump, had been a blur. His son told me that Sam had been confused and unable to participate in decisions about his care. The family had met with the doctors and concluded that Sam wouldn't want to go through open heart surgery. He did hope to live a little longer. And he wanted to spend whatever time he had—whether it was a month or a year or two—in his own apartment. He had had enough of hospitals.

Sam slept for twelve hours that night, and took two naps the next day. He didn't have the energy for physical therapy, and he was afraid that exertion would bring on that terrible crushing sensation in his chest. It was another three days before he felt ready to take a few tentative steps with the therapist. And then, when Sam was finally making progress, when the staff thought he was going to be going home soon, he had another bout of chest pain.

It came on suddenly, after dinner. The evening nurse took one look at Sam and called for an ambulance. She knew he had agreed he would not want cardiopulmonary resuscitation attempted and that the decision had been reached that he was not a candidate for bypass surgery. But he didn't have a "do not hospitalize" order. She didn't want him dying on her shift, and with his dusky color and thready pulse, he looked to her as if he just might be on his way out.

I got a call from the physician at the hospital the following day. He had nothing further to offer; Sam was already on five different kinds of medication for his heart. They had put him on a nitroglycerine drip and on heparin—continuous infusions of medication against chest pain and blood clots, respectively—but he couldn't stay on those indefinitely. They planned to "stabilize" him with the drugs by vein and then send him back.

I was in the transitional care unit when the burly ambulance drivers rolled him in the next day. Sam waved weakly. I thought I could see fear in his half smile, half grimace. I guessed that he was discouraged. When I was able to free up a good chunk of time to talk with him, I discovered he was also angry.

"At the hospital, they basically said they didn't understand why I was bothering them. If I wanted to live, I should have the bypass surgery. Since I wasn't going to have surgery, they figured I just wanted to be kept comfortable. Period."

"You do want to be comfortable," I elaborated, "but you also want simple things that might keep you going." He looked at me gratefully. "Such as the blood thinner and all your other heart medicines."

"Yes. One of the doctors seemed to think they should stop all those drips I was on and start a morphine drip instead. Just give me a lot of drugs and let me go."

"You're clearly not ready to go anywhere yet. And you don't need to be on continuous morphine. But a small amount of morphine when you get chest pain is not a bad idea."

Sam looked skeptical. "Morphine's what they give you when you're going to die."

"Not necessarily," I explained. "Morphine is an excellent cardiac drug—it's good against both chest pain and shortness of breath. It has effects on the blood vessels in much the same way that nitroglycerine does."[12]

It took some work convincing him, and the hospital physician's offer to use morphine as a form of "terminal sedation" didn't help.[13] But I argued that in the end, if Sam wanted an effective treatment for his chest pain, he needed to learn to take morphine. Moreover, going back and forth to the hospital wasn't the way he wanted to spend his time. The solution was to measure out a small amount of a concentrated form of liquid morphine which he could put under his tongue. The medicine would be absorbed quickly, just like an injection, but painlessly, without needles.

We began by using sublingual morphine, as it is called, in the transitional care unit whenever Sam developed chest pain. I explained to the nurses that they were not to ship Sam off to the hospital. I wrote out a protocol for using a few milligrams of morphine as soon as he felt a tightness in his chest. If the pain did not subside right away, he could get another dose fifteen minutes later.

At first, Sam was so nervous that he struggled to stay awake at night, convinced that he would wake up feeling like he had a massive stone on his chest, choking, with nothing available to help except a few drops of clear liquid under his tongue. For a week, Sam had no further chest pain, perhaps because his most strenuous activity was shaving. I thought that his last heart attack might have actually put an end to his pain: patients have pain when living tissue doesn't get enough oxygen, which in Sam's case resulted from severe narrowing of his main coronary artery. If the oxygen deficiency is severe enough, the heart muscle dies. At that point, the patient may have problems with the pumping function of the heart, or he may experience further chest pain if he develops narrowing in other blood vessels, but the original trouble spot won't bother him anymore.[14] But once Sam began doing more, buoyed by a week of pain-free existence, the pain returned. The transitional care unit was ready: the necessary morphine was available without delay, the nurse on duty understood the plan, and within minutes Sam started to feel better. The nurse insisted that a little improvement wasn't good enough—she gave him a second dose of medication and a little extra oxygen. The pain vanished.

Very slowly, Sam regained his confidence. He began working with the physical therapist, who taught him tricks for conserving his energy. He worked with a cognitive behavioral therapist, who showed him relaxation techniques. He spent time with his nurse learning to draw up a few milliliters of morphine in a syringe. After two weeks he announced that he was as good as he was going to get, and he was going home.

The facility social worker arranged for a visiting nurse to check on Sam three times a week and for a physical therapist to continue working with him at home. A home health aide came several times each week to help Sam shower, until he told her he didn't need her anymore.

Once in the next year Sam panicked when he couldn't breathe and called 911. The paramedics whisked him off to the emergency room, where the physicians were incredulous when he explained he'd been living by himself and took small amounts of morphine whenever he got chest pain. They weren't sure whether to refer him to the addiction service, believing him to be a drug addict, or to a psychiatrist, thinking he was delusional. Sam finally persuaded them to contact his cardiologist, who confirmed that Sam had had multiple heart attacks, had decided against bypass surgery, and wasn't a candidate for stent placement given the diffuse nature of his heart disease. And yes, for the most part he was able to treat his symptoms thanks to the judicious use of morphine along with several other newer and more expensive cardiac medicines. He probably would benefit from a shot of Lasix, a diuretic, the cardiologist suggested, and then they should send him home. No, the cardiologist reassured them, there was no need to see if he'd had another heart attack. The treatment would be the same, regardless.

Almost a year after I first met him in the transitional care unit, Sam's home health aide found him on the floor at home. He had collapsed in his bedroom while getting dressed, most likely from a fatal arrhythmia. I thought he had probably died instantly.

PHYSICIANS may cling to the notion that maximal medical treatment is the only viable option in acute illness, but they are gradually coming around to the view that a very different approach makes sense for treatment of chronic disease.[15] Chronic diseases are what make people frail. The frail person typically has impairments in multiple domains—for example, visual difficulties from macular degeneration, walking trouble from arthritis and peripheral vascular disease, and perhaps breathing difficulties from emphysema. He may manage reasonably well day-to-day, but because he has very limited reserves, a relatively minor illness such as influenza or a bladder infection can precipitate all sorts of trouble: he may develop chest pain from the increased stress on his heart, which may tip him into heart failure (causing fluid to back up into the lungs); or perhaps the infection will trigger acute confusion, impairing his judgment and leading to a fall and a broken hip. Treatment of acute problems in frail people is perilous because it often unmasks their underlying limited organ function.[16] Mildred Steiner was frail because of dementia and chronic cardiovascular disease; Sam Dryden was frail because of heart disease compounded by kidney and lung disease.

The usual approach to chronic disease is to try to prevent it and, when prevention fails, to go into rescue mode, heroically intervening to save patients from the brink of death. Prevention of heart disease, for instance, has revolved around treating high blood pressure and high cholesterol and exhorting patients to quit smoking cigarettes. These strategies paid off, with new cases of heart disease plummeting in the 1970s as compared with their all-time high in the previous decades. The number of heart attacks continued to fall in the 1980s.[17] Heart disease, however, remains the leading cause of death in older people, followed by cerebrovascular disease (various forms of stroke), which shares the same risk factors. A new approach to dealing with chronic disease that shows great promise is *disease management*, a strategy that involves ongoing monitoring of symptoms.[18]

Patients with congestive heart failure are prime candidates for the new disease management approach. Heart failure is a disorder in which the heart is weakened, leading to buildup of fluid in places it doesn't belong, such as the lungs. It is the leading cause of hospitalization in people over the age of 65. Slightly more than 5 million Americans suffer from congestive heart failure, of whom three-fourths are over the age of 65, and the cost of treating them in 2004 was close to $20 billion.[19] Standard American practice is to admit patients suffering from an exacerbation of heart failure to coronary care units—a phenomenon that occurs 800,000 times a year in Medicare patients—where they are closely monitored using technological interventions such as catheters that measure the pressure in the heart. Despite new and better treatments for congestive heart failure, it remains a devastating disease.

In light of these trends, the reports that started coming out of Australia in the late 1990s were quite startling. They demonstrated that a simple home-based intervention could dramatically affect the outcome of heart failure. The home-based approach consisted of a single visit one week after discharge from the hospital, made by a nurse and a pharmacist. This duo was charged with the responsibility of clarifying the prescribed medication regimen, detecting signs of impending relapse, and teaching caregivers what to watch out for. Interestingly, almost all the patients turned out to have a poor understanding of their disease and its treatment and, presumably as a result, about half of them were not taking their medications correctly. What was truly astonishing was that a single home visit led to a lower rate of readmission to the hospital, shorter hospital stays, lower costs, and fewer deaths. These results seemed too good to be true, but when the study was continued, first for eighteen months and then for four years, the patients seen at home consistently lived longer and were hospitalized less often than those receiving conventional care.[20]

Similar simple interventions were then tried in the United States and have been equally successful: for example, telephone calls made by a nurse to patients with congestive heart failure on a regular basis caused hospitalization rates and costs to plummet by 50 percent.[21] What is striking about these examples—and comparable strategies have been instituted for other chronic diseases—is that they do not involve *limiting* expensive care. They *do* entail adding disease management, a low-technology approach, to the treatment.

Disease management offers a successful way of addressing the most common diseases of old age in a labor-intensive rather than a technology-intensive way. It involves patients in their own care, not merely as partners in decision making, but as participants in treatment. It turns out that patients often do a better job than health care professionals. Monitoring the use of blood-thinning medication is a case in point.

Tens of thousands of older individuals take Warfarin, an anticoagulant, to prevent clots or strokes if they have an artificial heart valve, an irregular heart rhythm, or have previously had a blood clot. Taking Warfarin is a tricky business: the dose of the medication needs to be adjusted every few weeks—more often if the person starts a new medication such as an antibiotic. If the Warfarin dose is too high, it causes bleeding, and if it's too low, it offers no protection against all those ailments it was intended to prevent. Bleeding can mean a minor cut that just keeps on oozing, or it can involve a severe hemorrhage from a stomach ulcer or even bleeding into the brain after a fall. The most common and least effective means of monitoring Warfarin is by the physician: if a patient goes to his physician's office every few weeks, has a blood test done, and his physician then tells him what dose of medication to take, the amount of Warfarin in his system will be in the right range only some of the time. When the adjustment is done by an anticoagulation clinic, using a formal algorithm entered into a computer program, the percentage of the time that patients are in the therapeutic range rises and the risk of complications falls.[22] The highest success rates are achieved when patients adjust their own Warfarin doses using a small machine to check their blood levels, following a set of rules for how to alter the dose.[23] While this is arguably a strategy best suited to the educated, middle-class patient, it may work better in less well-educated patients than the current system, which requires traveling to the physician's office or the lab and relies on telephone messages or postcards for dosage adjustment.

Disease management programs also make use of nurses, particularly the more highly skilled nurse practitioners, and physician assistants in novel ways. Instead of performing tasks which physicians used to do but which do not require the extensive knowledge and training of an M.D., these clinicians take on roles that no one currently fills in the conventional medical model. The nurse practitioner establishes a relationship with a patient and is available by phone to guide patients through the frequent minor crises which, if not dealt with in a timely fashion, can result in major disease flares. If need be, the nurse practitioner will make a home visit, but typically she can gather sufficient information from the patient, who takes his own pulse and weighs himself, to advise on medication adjustment.[24]

Nurses are far better suited than physicians to talking about options. It is no coincidence that the Study to Understand Prognoses and Preferences for Care (SUPPORT) relied on nurses to talk to seriously ill, hospitalized patients about their prognosis and preferences for care. The hope was that if both patients and doctors had information about prognosis and patients' values and if the communication between patients and physicians were enhanced, then doctors would honor their patients' wishes. The Evercare program, a model HMO providing nursing home care, employs nurse practitioners to deliver the bulk of the medical care and to talk to patients and families about limitations of care. As a result of these discussions, families are far more likely to accept treatment in the nursing home rather than transfer to the hospital whenever their relative becomes ill.

Disease management can abort the cycle of disease exacerbations that precipitate a trip to the emergency room, lead to hospitalization, and then culminate in deconditioning. By involving patients in their own care in new ways, it also prepares them to raise the issue of intermediate care when they develop an acute illness. Physicians are catching on to the fact that disease management works, and Medicare, for the first time, is funding chronic care improvement programs.[25] But the impetus for further change will need to come from patients and their families. In general, the consumer movement has been a potent stimulus to reforming medical practice. The move from anesthetized childbirth to natural childbirth and the shift from radical mastectomies to simple mastectomies (and now to lumpectomies) for breast cancer testify to the power of the consumer. The baby boomers are the ultimate consumerists, not shy about demanding what we feel is our due. The challenge for this group, once we become frail, is to come to regard "our due" not as more and more high-tech medicine, but as intermediate care. The role we will play as disease managers will not only expose us to another strand of medicine, it will also put us in contact with nurse practitioners who can serve as our allies in the quest for intermediate care.

THREE

Doing the Right Thing Near the End

OVERTREATMENT, or at least providing too much of the wrong treatment and not enough of the right stuff, is commonplace in American medicine. It is going to be an increasing problem as the baby boomers age if robust elders demand screening tests that are worse than useless and if frail elders insist on subjecting their vulnerable bodies to the assaults of maximally aggressive medicine. But the potential to cause needless pain and suffering while simultaneously breaking the bank is at its greatest as we get closer to the very end of life. The temptation to keep on fighting, to summon the heavy artillery, is enormous when death is the alternative. The truth is that at the very end of life, death is no longer an "alternative"—a locution that suggests there is another possibility. Death is the only possible outcome. What we can control is not whether or not we die, but the style in which we do it.

SADIE SOLOMON was 90 years old and suffered from advanced Alzheimer's disease. Her daughters did not accept that she was dying. Or rather, they believed it was their obligation—and that of the physicians and nurses who cared for Sadie in the nursing home—to keep her alive, whatever it took.

Sadie had difficulty swallowing solid food, and she had little interest in the pureed concoctions, puddings, and ice creams the dietician ordered for her instead. For over a year, she had subsisted on high-calorie protein drinks. Ultimately, she began having difficulty swallowing liquids as well as solids. One stormy November day, some of her strawberry milk shake went into her windpipe and traveled to her lungs. Within 24 hours, Sadie came down with a full-blown pneumonia. She was breathing rapidly, she was feverish, and she was only barely conscious.

Pneumonia, in the words of a wise physician in the 1890s, is or at least can be the old person's best friend.[1] Everyone has to die of something, and infection is often what turns a potentially protracted course of decline and disability into a brief terminal illness. I recommended that the nurses keep Sadie comfortable by giving her oxygen for her breathlessness, Tylenol for her fever, and morphine for chest pain. But Sadie's daughters did not regard comfort as the major goal of care. On the basis of their personal religious convictions, they felt the overriding goal should be the prolongation of their mother's life. With some reluctance, I agreed to insert an intravenous catheter and to administer fluids and antibiotics.

Sadie improved transiently—her temperature went down, she stopped gasping for breath, and she became more alert. She returned to her baseline mute state, her emaciated body permanently bent at the hips and knees. Within a week of her completing a course of antibiotics, the process recurred. I met with Sadie's daughters to explain that patients dying of Alzheimer's disease are prone to repeated bouts of pneumonia. Nothing could reverse the underlying, inexorable progression toward death. Treatment of the pneumonia and dehydration, while potentially able to prolong life temporarily, could not interrupt the cycle.

Not only was Sadie dying, she was also suffering. She coughed, she was hot, and she struggled to catch her breath. Our therapy for her pneumonia added to her suffering: we performed blood tests, I tried repeatedly to insert an intravenous catheter into her wayward veins, and the nurses tied her down to try to prevent her from removing it once I had secured it. I strongly recommended that we switch to a palliative approach to care, and Sadie's nurse and social worker agreed. By palliation I meant oxygen and Tylenol, but no needles, no restraints, and no antibiotics.

Sadie's daughters felt equally strongly that they wanted their mother's life prolonged. Suffering, they said, was of little consequence compared to the immeasurable value of life itself. They were adamant that we should deliver whatever curative treatments were medically indicated—not only the intravenous fluids and antibiotics and oxygen that I had ordered, but also, if technically advisable, a respirator for breathing, available only in a hospital. They acknowledged that Sadie had never expressed any interest in being kept alive this way and had not herself been religious.

For the third time in a month, Sadie developed pneumonia. She gasped for breath. Her lips turned blue. She wore an oxygen mask—this time she was so weak and tired that she did not have the strength to pull it off—but the oxygen could not penetrate the viscous secretions that blocked her air passages. The nurses and nurses' aides taking care of Sadie, who were very attached to her and saw themselves as a second family, pleaded with me to prescribe morphine to alleviate her anxiety and her physical distress.

Instead, at the family's request, I transferred Sadie to a nearby acute care hospital, where the emergency room physician put a breathing tube down her throat, hooked her up to a respirator, and admitted her to the intensive care unit (ICU). While she was in the hospital, she had a heart attack and a stress ulcer. For three days she remained in the ICU, where she was both physically restrained and pharmacologically sedated to prevent her from removing her tubes. She received blood transfusions and several liters of intravenous fluid, much of which leaked into her arms and legs, which consequently ballooned to twice their usual size. As soon as she was medically stable, the hospital physicians transferred her back to the nursing home, a nasogastric tube dangling from her nose. She died in her sleep a few days later.

Sadie's daughters invoked their religious beliefs as the reason for insisting on all possible interventions for their mother. In fact, religious traditions generally understand that mortality is part of the human condition, that death is inevitable, and that it is wrong to cause suffering when a person is facing death. In Catholicism, for instance, widely regarded as a "right to life" tradition, the presumption is to favor life, but in treating dying patients, physicians are told to weigh the benefits and burdens of those treatments. The National Conference of Catholic Bishops goes so far as to endorse a family or community perspective, arguing that treatment can be forgone if the burden to the patient's family or to the surrounding community is excessive. Their directive on health care starts by asserting that "a person has a moral obligation to use ordinary or proportionate means of preserving life" but then explains that "proportionate means are those that in the judgment of the patient offer a reasonable hope of benefit and do not entail an excessive burden or impose excessive expense on the family or the community." With respect to the issue of artificial nutrition, the Bishops acknowledge that "there should be a presumption in favor of providing nutrition and hydration to all patients, including patients who require medically assisted nutrition and hydration, as long as this is of sufficient benefit to outweigh the burdens involved to the patient."[2]

Orthodox Jewish thinkers, while far more heterogeneous than their Catholic counterparts, have similarly regarded dying patients as distinct from patients who can potentially be cured. The major talmudic teaching on this point is based, as is much of traditional Judaism, on a story. Rabbi Judah the Prince, a teacher revered by his students, lay dying. In the pre-narcotic era of the third century, when the story took place, he had no medication available and was in excruciating pain. His followers prayed fervently for his life, and as long as they kept praying, according to tradition, he continued to live. Rabbi Judah's maid saw how much he was suffering and pleaded for the followers to stop their prayers and allow the rabbi to die. Convinced they were doing the right thing, they ignored her. Finally, the maid decided to take matters into her own hands. She climbed to the roof and began hurling dishes and pots to the ground. When the stoneware hit

the ground, making a terrific din, the assembled group momen-
tarily stopped praying. During that instant, according to the legend, the rabbi died and his soul departed. The Talmud comments
on the "wisdom" of the maidservant, who recognized that it is
wrong to try to prevent death when it is inevitable.[3]

Traditional Judaism also explicitly views intractable suffering
as a reason not to prolong life. The major talmudic text dealing
with this situation is another story, the disturbing tale of Rabbi
Chanina, who was burned alive by the Romans for teaching the
Jewish bible. The Romans, known for their sophistication in torture, ordered his executioner to cover the rabbi with wet sponges.
The idea was that the water would slow the victim's death and
prolong his agony. The executioner, recognizing that Rabbi Chanina's death was certain and seeing his extraordinary suffering,
refused. According to the Talmud, the executioner then threw
himself into the flames as an act of contrition, and a voice from
heaven announced that both the Rabbi and the executioner had a
place in the world to come.[4] The talmudic rabbis applauded the
executioner's behavior, giving rise to the view that there is no obligation to prolong the life of a dying person who is suffering. Of
course, it is problematic to infer anything about how physicians
should care for the dying from this story of Roman torture. But
perhaps the best reason for believing that this gruesome story
teaches compassion for those who are suffering and dying is its
treatment of the executioner. If the Roman carrying out his government's fiendish death penalty is behaving morally by ever so
slightly shortening life in the service of diminishing pain, then
surely the physician who fails to prolong life with aggressive interventions that only prolong suffering is at least as moral.

Sadie's daughters were offered a different interpretation by their religious advisers; they were told that their tradition required any and all potentially life-saving interventions. They were not apprised that even religions that emphasize the sanctity of life also acknowledge the inevitability of death.

It was exactly this sort of case that made physicians begin invoking "futility" as a reason for withholding aggressive treatment. Futility became a hot topic in the late 1980s, as physicians struggled over the issue of whether they could unilaterally refuse medical interventions they believed were ineffective.[5] Physicians hoped to be able to assert definitively that certain disputed treatments were physiologically futile, and would have been delighted to find a technical solution to the question of what constituted appropriate treatment for a variety of often fatal clinical conditions. An intervention was clearly futile if it made no biomedical sense. Antibiotics, for example, are a futile treatment for viral illnesses because they work by targeting a stage of the bacterial life cycle and are ineffective in killing viruses. Similarly, laetrile, a once popular "alternative" remedy for cancer, is physiologically futile because there is no scientific evidence that it has any effect on cancer cells.

Although it is relatively easy to label a treatment that cannot possibly work as futile, it's a lot harder to figure out how to classify a treatment that could theoretically work, but rarely does. Several medical ethicists concluded that futility is most fruitfully regarded as a statistical concept: if a treatment has failed in 100 consecutive, similar cases, then the treatment should be viewed as futile.[6] The problem with this definition is putting it into practice. Who is keeping count of how many older people fail to survive an intervention such as cardiopulmonary resuscitation? How similar do the patients have to be for us to consider them comparable? If we look at the results of attempted CPR in five different institutions, each trying and failing to resuscitate twenty patients, can we conclude the success rate is less than 1/100, just because it was 0/20 five times? The personnel, the available equipment, and various other circumstances were somewhat different in the five institutions. And finally, suppose the treatment *does* work in 1 out of 100 cases. The treatment is then clearly not impossible, it is not physically nonsensical, but is a 1 percent chance good enough to subject 99 people to an ineffective intervention for the sake of the one person in whom it would work?[7] And just what does "work" mean? Survive for a few hours? Live long enough to be discharged from the hospital? Make it for six months?

Mistakenly believing that the courts would be willing to let physicians define futility, Hennepin County Hospital in Minneapolis, Minnesota, petitioned the court to appoint a new surrogate decision maker for its patient, Helga Wanglie. Mrs. Wanglie was an 88-year-old woman who developed multiple complications after hip surgery, culminating in a coma. She was kept alive in the ICU of Hennepin County Hospital on a ventilator. The hospital wanted to have the patient's husband removed as surrogate decision maker because he favored continued use of a ventilator to help keep her alive. To Mr. Wanglie, the prospect of continued life was sufficient justification to maintain his wife on a ventilator, regardless of the probability of her regaining consciousness. To the hospital staff, keeping Mrs. Wanglie's heart and lungs going without any evidence of consciousness, and with no expectation that she would ever regain consciousness, was not a benefit at all. At issue was not the technical consideration of whether the ventilator was effective in supporting life; rather, the question was just what purpose the ventilator served—simply to maintain the circulation? or to restore the patient to a basic level of thinking, acting life? The court restricted its decision to the narrow question of whether Mr. Wanglie could serve as his wife's health care proxy, or whether he should be replaced by a court-appointed surrogate. Since there was no reason to disqualify Mr. Wanglie, other than his refusal to authorize the hospital to re-move life support, he remained the substitute decision maker. The court ignored the question of whether there could be legiti-mate limits on what decisions he was entitled to make.[8]

Attempts to resolve the futility debate met a similar fate in bioethical circles as they did in the courts. Futility came to be seen by some as too elusive to be a helpful concept, and by others as a front for rationing. In the Wanglie case, some ethicists argued that the "real" reason the hospital wanted to withdraw the venti-lator was that the cost of her care had already exceeded $800,000.[9] The hospital countered that Helga belonged to a health mainte-nance organization, which professed to be perfectly willing to pay all her expenses. The rejoinder was that even if the hospital did not suffer financially, Helga was taking up an ICU bed and was potentially depriving a more "viable" patient of a scarce resource. The net result of the first round of debates was that the American Medical Association (AMA) accorded the concept of futility a "do-not-resuscitate" status, stating: "a fully objective and concrete definition of futility is unattainable." The AMA exhorted physicians and patients to resolve their differences by improved com-munication and, if necessary, by calling in an ethics committee or other neutral party.[10]

Despite the grim prognosis for "futility" as a concept, it has failed to disappear as a concern for physicians and nurses. The reason is that negotiation and mediation do not always work. When neither side is willing to compromise, these measures fail. And medical personnel have been unwilling to compromise when they believe the treatment they are asked to administer is morally wrong. The reasons for believing that some interventions are wrong go beyond ineffectiveness and beyond costliness. Physi-cians balk at providing treatment that is very unlikely to succeed in prolonging life *and* that causes pain and suffering to the pa-tient *and* that is expensive *and* that is undertaken in a patient who was near the end of life before the acute problem developed. Sadie is an excellent example: even before she started having recurrent bouts of pneumonias, she was in the final stage of Alzheimer's disease, an invariably fatal condition. Hospital care was very un-likely to prolong her life; a number of studies have found that the majority of patients with advanced dementia who are hospital-ized with pneumonia are dead within six months, regardless of how aggressively they are treated.[11] Sadie showed signs of suffer-ing as a result of her treatment: she moaned, she cried, and she tried to remove the assorted tubes that were inserted into most of her bodily orifices. Finally, the cost of her ICU stay exceeded $2000 per day—and the total cost of care like Sadie's, intensive care in very old people that is followed by death, is estimated to be over $15 billion per year.[12]

In Sadie Solomon's case, all four factors were present—low effectiveness, high burden, high cost, and imminent death. The more factors that apply in a given situation, the more objectionable is the treatment. If, for example, a treatment is expensive and is able at best to maintain a patient in a persistent vegetative state, I would say this treatment is unfortunate and undesirable, but not nearly as objectionable as a similar treatment that also causes suffering. Between 10,000 and 25,000 adult patients in the United States languish in a persistent vegetative state today, only some of whom are elderly.[13] These individuals are able to breathe on their own, but their level of awareness is so profoundly diminished that they are not able to experience anything, let alone to communicate. They are sometimes described as being in a state of "coma with eyes open." Since they often have no medical problem other than their disturbed brain function, they can be kept alive for extended periods (in many cases for years) with good nursing care (for example, turning them from side to side to avoid skin breakdown) and with artificial nutrition and hydration. Is it wise to keep these patients alive, patients who will never wake up and speak or move deliberately or experience sensation?

The right-to-life position is that all life is precious and should be preserved. The counter-argument is that respecting life should not entail treating someone who has lost all his human capacities the same way we treat someone who experiences pain and pleasure. Likewise, it is no affirmation of the sanctity of life to confuse someone who is dead with someone who is alive. While it seems to me that pumping nutrients into patients simply to keep their hearts going is both foolish and a waste of valuable resources, it bothers me a great deal less than does Sadie's treatment: Sadie was able to feel pain—her moans, her grimaces, and her expressive eye movements in response to painful stimuli made that eminently clear—but individuals in a persistent vegetative state cannot.

Similarly, treatments that are medically of little value but are inexpensive are far less disturbing than are costly treatments. Physicians routinely give antibiotics to nursing home patients with dementia when they develop a fever, although at least one study found that such patients are just as likely to die with antibiotics as without them.[14] Many nursing home patients with fevers have viral infections, which do not respond to antibiotics but which may resolve on their own. And even those individuals with advanced dementia who have bacterial infections are likely to die whether or not they are vigorously treated with antibiotics: their ability to fight off infection is severely limited. But if families and physicians feel more comfortable administering what *might* be an effective treatment—antibiotics for pneumonia or a bladder infection—and if the patient is able to swallow the pills, the potentially "futile" expenditure of $100 does not strike me as outrageous. If the patient cannot swallow and has to get the probably useless antibiotic by vein, as happened with Sadie, and if she is alert enough to find the insertion of the needle painful, then the treatment starts to become more troublesome. And if the patient has no accessible veins and has to have a special catheter inserted directly into a large vein near the heart, an intervention that is associated with a risk of puncturing the lung, then the burdens even more clearly outweigh the benefits.

The likelihood of benefit and the imminence of death are also relevant. Patients with advanced dementia often become dehydrated because most of them don't experience thirst. Giving fluids by vein typically corrects the dehydration. It does not fix the underlying problem that predisposed them to dehydration in the first place, their dementia, which will ultimately result in death. But doctors can at least transiently reverse the lethargy, the low blood pressure, and the biochemical abnormalities that are the hallmarks of dehydration. I often recommend keeping such patients comfortable with ice chips rather than subjecting them to technological fixes, since "fixing" dehydration simply allows the patient to have it again or to develop pneumonia or a pressure ulcer in the immediate future. But I do not think it's wrong to treat the dehydration. If the treatment is painful or distressing—for example, if the patient has to be hospitalized for placement of a gastrostomy tube (a tube inserted into the stomach through which fluid and nutrients can be supplied)—then the intervention becomes objectionable. But the use of fluid for hydration seems far more reasonable than, say, the widespread practice of prescribing cancer chemotherapy with many side effects for a very debilitated patient when the therapy has only a 10 percent success rate in far more vigorous patients.

Finally, in thinking about how much suffering and how much expense to tolerate, it matters whether death is truly imminent. The reason Sadie's caregivers found her treatment unconscionable was that her prognosis was abysmal regardless of what was done. To inflict suffering on a woman who was clearly at the end of her life in the hope of eking out a few more hours, days, or even weeks seemed unjustified.

As long as we continue to offer treatments, even if they are rarely effective, invasive, and costly, there will be patients (or family members) who will opt for those treatments. They may do so because they believe that if a treatment is considered, it must have some degree of efficacy. They may do so because they subscribe to magical thinking and are convinced that whatever the odds of survival, they or their parent will be the one in a million who survives. They may do so because they come from a culture in which authority figures, including physicians, routinely try to deprive them of useful services. The only way to ensure that such patients are not subjected to inappropriate treatments is either to have a futility policy or to limit third-party coverage for such care.

Futility policies exist at both the institutional and the community level. A relatively simple, very narrow futility policy is the "CPR not indicated" policy found in a number of hospitals. These institutions lay out a set of circumstances in which a physician can decide not to perform CPR if a patient's heart stops and he isn't breathing. Typically, the situation is that the patient is dying, for example of widespread cancer, and a second physician confirms that death is expected within days. The primary care doctor can then write the order "CPR not indicated."[15] In one well-publicized case the physicians did exactly that, the patient died, CPR was not attempted, and the family sued. The physicians were exonerated in court.[16] This was a jury trial, not a judge's ruling, but it is striking that when the doctors explained why they believed CPR was not indicated, their decision was upheld. Problems seem to arise if the hospital goes to court while the patient is still alive and requests permission to withhold treatment on the grounds of futility. In those instances, courts regularly insist that physicians defer to patients or their surrogates for decisions about how much and what kind of care to administer.[17]

Broader than institutional policies are community futility policies. Institutional futility guidelines have their place—they allow hospitals or nursing homes to specify the kinds of treatment that are consistent with their particular philosophy. A patient seeking an abortion knows perfectly well that she cannot expect to have it performed at a Catholic hospital. Some Alzheimer's special care units state that their philosophy is to focus primarily on a resident's comfort and that they do not offer intravenous therapy, feeding tubes, or transfer to an acute hospital. They describe their approach up front, which allows prospective residents and their families to select a facility with a compatible philosophy. The assumption is that in a pluralistic society, there will be many institutions that espouse varying perspectives on the kind of care they provide. Community futility policies go further: they take as their starting point the idea that there are certain treatments, in particular situations, that violate the generally held view of appropriate care. To the extent that individuals of differing socioeconomic backgrounds, varying ethnic groups, and assorted occupations concur on such a standard, it represents a *reasonable* standard.

Several communities have come up with exactly this kind of futility guideline. The Colorado Collective for Medical Decisions, a grassroots coalition in Denver, created separate task forces in areas ranging from adult intensive care to neonatal intensive care. The groups were charged with enumerating particular treatments that the members agreed were unacceptable. Once the task force agreed on its list of inappropriate treatments, it forwarded its recommendations to a larger group of community representatives for their feedback. This give-and-take resulted in a true consensus document which could then be used by health care institutions throughout the Denver area.[18] The medical task forces all came up with specific guidelines. For example, the adult intensive care subcommittee agreed that ICU care is not recommended for patients in a persistent vegetative state and that CPR is not recommended in a variety of situations, including end-stage dementia and persistent vegetative state.[19]

A different approach was developed in Houston. Representatives from multiple institutions in Texas drew up a draft of guidelines that was submitted to participating institutions for comment. Included were teaching and non-teaching hospitals, for-profit and not-for-profit hospitals, public and private institutions, and secular and religious facilities. The task force synthesized these comments into a revised document entitled "Guidelines on Institutional Policies on the Determination of Medically Inappropriate Interventions." The key features of the policy are that patients or their surrogates must be involved in decision making, that physicians must not act unilaterally, and that an interdisciplinary review process will handle disputes. When disputes cannot be resolved, transfer to another facility will be discussed; if this is impossible or impractical, the Houston policy allows discontinuation or withholding of the intervention in question, but insists that other medically appropriate care for the patient be continued. The guidelines were supported by most of the major hospitals in the greater Houston area, but only three institutions approved them for use.[20]

Unfortunately, there is little information about whether anyone actually adheres to community futility policies. The Denver Collaborative no longer exists, and a number of the task forces never completed their work. Houston developed a community policy that was incorporated into the "policies and procedures" of area hospitals, but it is unclear whether physicians or administrators working in those institutions are familiar with its content. California and Florida also developed policies of uncertain effectiveness.[21]

We do know that institutional futility policies are rarely followed. One study of a "CPR not indicated" policy at two university-affiliated hospitals found that interns routinely misunderstood both the intent and the specifics of the policy.[22] An informal survey of house officers at the acute care hospital with which I was previously affiliated indicated that most doctors did not know that such a policy existed, and those who did know had no idea what medical conditions were covered or what they needed to do to support writing a "CPR not indicated" order.

The difficulty in developing policies and the widespread lack of knowledge about those that manage to come into being are not entirely surprising. Finding common ground in the medical ethics arena is hard but not impossible, as the members of the National Commission for the Protection of Human Subjects of Biomedical and Behavioral Research discovered. The key to their success, as related by one of the staff members, was the recognition that they didn't have to agree on the reason for their recommendations; they merely had to agree on the recommendations. If they started with principles, they became hopelessly tangled up in their disparate perspectives. If they focused exclusively on what they believed to be right, they discovered a surprising degree of uniformity.[23] But for this group to come to any conclusions, they needed a mandate to formulate a position, and they needed support to continue their work.

It's also not surprising that those futility guidelines which, against all odds, are in fact produced, are often ignored. Most clinical practice guidelines, regardless of the topic, are ignored or forgotten. Professionals are much better at devising recommendations than they are at implementing them. Good processes for designing guidelines include the involvement of the people who will eventually be called upon to implement the recommendations. If the very people who are expected to prescribe pain medication draw up the list of what medications should be used, under what circumstances, and in what doses, they are more likely to buy into the finished product. The trouble is that those same physicians forget, or move to new positions, or are joined by other doctors who were not involved in writing the guidelines. Study after study demonstrates that practice guidelines are not followed—unless there is a continuing educational process to remind physicians of their contents, or a feedback process to reward those who abide by the guidelines and to criticize those who do not.

Even when physicians do know what the official recommendations are—administering beta-blockers and aspirin in patients who have had a myocardial infarction, for example—they are remarkably adept at finding excuses for why their particular patients should be exceptions to the rule. And of course sometimes the patients *do* constitute exceptions; for instance, the guidelines for optimal therapy typically mean optimal life-prolonging therapy, whereas a given patient might be more interested in optimal comfort-promoting therapy.

Guidelines are also problematic because different professional societies often come up with mutually contradictory practice guidelines, leaving the individual physician completely uncertain as to the "right" course of action. There are, for example, multiple competing sets of recommendations for periodic screening: the U.S. Preventive Services Task Force has one set and the Canadian Task Force has another. They do not always concur, and in those instances where they do, still other professional organizations such as the American Cancer Society or the American Heart Association often weigh in with a contrary opinion. If there is little uniformity when it comes to evidence-based medicine, we can expect even less homogeneity in a value-laden arena such as futility.

Even when we have a single guideline and its contents are widely disseminated and physicians generally agree with its recommendations, there will still be difficulty with implementation.[24] The problem arises when physicians inform patients of an available treatment and then turn around and say it is not recommended. Some patients will go along with their doctor's recommendations; others will suspect they are being deprived of a beneficial treatment by some anonymous authority. Far more logical would be to tie the guidelines to Medicare reimbursement. If the guidelines support use of the treatment, Medicare will pay for it; if they don't recommend the treatment, Medicare won't cover it.

If patients insist on a non-covered treatment and can find a doctor willing to provide it, they can have the treatment—provided they are willing to pay for it.

Many treatments suddenly become far less desirable when patients have to pay out of pocket. The study of attitudes toward screening tests that I described in Chapter 1 reveals that patients may "want" a variety of tests even if they have not been shown to be effective, but when asked how much they would be willing to pay for those tests, they indicated that if the test cost more than $15 or $20, it would not be nearly so attractive. Similarly, I suspect that ICU care at $2000 per day would be a good deal less appealing than it is now if families could not rely on Medicare to cover the cost (after a deductible, which they would have had to pay even for non-ICU care). For those who protest that rationing on the basis of ability to pay is unjust, I share that perspective for *useful* treatment. For useless, painful, and costly care, I am less concerned about inequities. Under such a system, only the affluent will have the opportunity to torment their dying relatives. We need to begin by defining a range of acceptable end-of-life treatments, using the consensus approach of the National Institutes of Health, and then restrict Medicare reimbursement to those treatments that meet the new standard.

Discussions of futility will fade away once we give patients what they need and do not merely discuss depriving them of what they don't need. These problems will begin to dissipate when we start doing a better job of informing patients about their prognosis, and when patients, their families, and their religious advisers develop a deeper appreciation of the limits of medicine. Paradoxically, the same excessive focus on individual choice that is part of the reason why physicians routinely receive and honor requests for futile therapy also leads to requests for accelerated death through physician-assisted suicide.

Physician-assisted suicide (PAS) is a sanitized way of saying killing oneself with a physician's help.[25] It is the ultimate form of control—controlling the time and manner of one's own death. PAS leaves the final step to the patient himself rather than granting to physicians the authority to deliberately and explicitly end a patient's life. In Oregon, the one state where PAS is legal, the procedure is carefully regulated and involves several steps. The patient must be terminally ill—and must have a second opinion to confirm the prognosis. He must twice request a prescription for medication with which to commit suicide. After a 15-day waiting period, the primary physician may write a prescription, usually for phenobarbital. The patient can then take a lethal dose of pills, if he decides his life is truly unbearable.

In the first year when PAS was legal in Oregon, only 23 patients went through this procedure to obtain a prescription. Only 15 actually took the medication. Six patients died from their underlying disease, and two were still alive at the end of the year. In the second year, the number increased very slightly to 33 out of a total of nearly 7,000 deaths, where it leveled off.[26] What the small numbers suggest is that what people really want is to die well. They want a dignified death; they want to be free of pain; and they do not want to be a burden on those they love.[27]

WHEN I was doing office-based geriatric consultation, I evaluated Jay Robinson, a 66-year-old recently retired engineer who came in at the insistence of his two daughters. Their father, they

reported, who had always been able to do complicated calcula-
tions in his head, now had trouble figuring out how much of a tip
to leave when they went out to a restaurant. In other respects, he
seemed to be his usual self—at least most of the time. His daughter Alexandra thought he had slowed down and noticed that his
thinking was sometimes a little fuzzy. Normally a very precise
man, he had trouble finding words. He had difficulty making decisions. His wife discovered him staring into his closet, seemingly
deliberating on what shirt to wear, and still undecided ten minutes later—even though all the shirts he was gazing at were virtually indistinguishable.

His daughter Jeanette worried that he was depressed. He had
worked 10-hour days for forty years, ever since he had received a
master's degree in engineering, and though he was devoted to his
family and enjoyed reading an occasional mystery novel or going
to the movies, he had never cultivated any hobbies. Work had
been the fulcrum of his existence, and Jeanette was worried that
he would fall apart without it. She had urged her father to continue as a consultant with his firm and had been puzzled when he
told her he didn't think he would be able to concentrate.

Alexandra, the younger daughter, was afraid that her father was
developing Alzheimer's disease. The reason he had been so intent
on retiring at age 65 was that he could no longer do the work, she
thought. Alexandra had noticed subtle changes in her father a
year earlier. He seemed to have difficulty with simple things such
as tying his shoes. He could not remember telephone numbers—
and they had always called him a walking phone book. Alexandra
had seen a television program about Alzheimer's disease and was
convinced that her father showed all the signs of dementia.

Mrs. Robinson was a quiet, passive woman. At first she denied that anything was wrong, but when her husband went into the examination room to undress, she broke down in tears. He had given his whole life to the company, she cried. Now that he had retired and could finally enjoy his family and perhaps take her on the trip to China she had always dreamed of, he had suddenly become "possessed."

Mr. Robinson's neurological examination was markedly abnormal. He could not copy a simple design; his movements were clumsy; and, what was most striking, he could not count. He also had trouble with his memory and with language. This did not look like depression to me, and the rapid onset of multiple deficits argued against Alzheimer's. I ordered a CT scan and arranged for the family to return in a week, after I received the results.

Jay Robinson had a very large brain tumor. The location and configuration strongly suggested the most rapidly lethal of the various types of malignant brain tumors, a glioblastoma.

On Mr. Robinson's next visit, after he had had a confirmatory brain biopsy and a consultation with a neuro-oncologist, I observed that he had deteriorated markedly. He was unable to articulate a complete sentence. He did not appear to recognize the members of his family. He clearly regarded them as benevolent figures, but I was not sure he knew their positions in the family, and he certainly could not remember their names. And this previously dignified, well-spoken man drooled.

Jeanette explained that the neuro-oncologist had suggested surgery and chemotherapy. Together, these interventions might prolong her father's life by a few months. Much of that time he would spend in a hospital, whether as an inpatient recovering from the operation, or in a rehab facility trying to get back on his feet, or in the outpatient department to receive intravenous chemotherapy. The doctor would not promise any improvement in his mental status, although he thought it probably would get better, for a limited time, before it got much worse. The reason they had made an appointment to see me was that the family agreed that surgery and chemo were out. Mr. Robinson had told them he would not want to live this way. They wanted to know whether I could give him something to end it all.[28]

I looked at their faces. Jeanette was imploring. Her sister was crying quietly. Her mother was gazing ahead, stony-faced. Jay Robinson was playing with the buttons on his sweater. He no longer had the dexterity to open or close them, so he just pulled at them, starting at the top and working his way down, and then going back up to the first one.

"What is it you are most afraid of?" I asked.

There were a lot of things. Jeanette worried that her father would be unable to walk to the bathroom and would become incontinent. He was a very proud and private man and would never have wanted to rely on others for such basic personal care. Alexandra was worried about her mother—she didn't think her mother had the stamina or the physical strength to take care of her father, who was six feet tall and weighed 180 pounds, though he was rapidly losing weight. Mrs. Robinson had heard that people with brain tumors sometimes developed hallucinations. She could bear the physical weakness, she said, but she didn't want to see her husband "go crazy." And they were all afraid that when he couldn't swallow pills anymore and therefore could not take his anti-seizure medication, he would have horrible seizures.

The Robinsons were concerned about Jay's loss of dignity and about his suffering. Very gently, I told them there were ways to address those concerns without resorting to euthanasia. They were skeptical. They had looked at their husband and father and had seen devastation. It was not going to get any better. They were not sure they could face what was coming.

I told them that if they were certain that aggressive treatment was out of the question—and they were—the best approach was to enroll in a hospice program. The goal would be to keep Jay at home, out of ambulances, out of hospitals, and enable him to die with as much dignity and as little pain as possible. He would be assigned a hospice nurse who would visit him at home and would suggest adjustments of his medications. The hospice would provide the medicines as well as a hospital bed, a commode, and whatever other equipment was needed so that he could be cared for at home.

I looked at Jay Robinson, who was quiet now, staring in my general direction without showing signs of actually seeing me. His face was gaunt, his belt on the last hole, barely holding up his now baggy pants. "I don't think he has much time left," I said softly.

They wanted to know what the end would be like. They felt they had to be sure it would not be a nightmare, totally beyond their control. I said that when he stopped taking the steroids, the medication that was used to decrease the swelling around his brain, he would probably lapse into unconsciousness fairly quickly. If he no longer took liquids by mouth, he would become dehydrated, and that would also push him into a coma. If there were any seizures, he could be given rectal suppositories to stop them. There would be no need for intravenous fluids or medications. All his care would focus on his comfort. If they wished, I would serve as the physician who worked with the hospice team to direct his care.

Jay Robinson died two weeks later. He had lost interest in food and drink. His fluid intake had become erratic, and he had developed lethargy. Because he was sleepy all the time, he stopped being able to take his medications and became even drowsier. One day he went to sleep and never woke up again. In his last hours, his breathing was labored and he seemed to be bothered by thick secretions from his lungs, so I ordered medications in the form of a skin patch to ease his breathing and to dry up the secretions. His daughters were holding his hands when he took his last breath.

Patients may have different ideas about what dying well means, though they typically agree that they want a dignified death, they would like to be free of pain, and they do not want to be a burden on those they love. Having control over the dying process, which is what physician-assisted suicide (PAS) is all about, is rarely an end; it is a means. By focusing on the means, advocates of PAS lose sight of their true objective. The emphasis should be on ensuring that patients can and do receive prescriptions for appropriate pain medications, not that they have access to prescriptions for suicide. And the emphasis should be on legislating support for hospice care, not debating PAS.

Modern hospice care was born in 1967, when Dame Cicely Saunders founded St. Christopher's Hospice in London. Her goal was to provide excellent symptomatic treatment for dying patients. Her insight was that patients who are not receiving curative treatment still deserve and need some kind of treatment. Just because certain interventions are not appropriate or desired or just don't work, this does not mean that *no* medical interventions are warranted. Dying patients are prone to anxiety, depression, and confusion, symptoms that can be treated with traditional medical solutions such as pills, oxygen, and injections. Moreover, expertise is required to manage these symptoms effectively—to treat pain without causing excessive sedation and to guard against other side effects such as constipation and hallucinations.

Dame Cicely says she was inspired to create a model—and novel—way to care for the terminally ill through her conversations with David Tasma, a young Polish Jew who was dying of inoperable cancer when she met him in a British hospital in 1947. Saunders was, at the time, what was quaintly referred to as a "lady almoner," something like a medical social worker. The two talked about how ill-suited a busy hospital ward was to controlling pain and coming to terms with death. Tasma had survived the Warsaw ghetto only to succumb to cancer at age 40. In his will, he left 500 pounds to Saunders with the message: "I will be a window in your home."[29] She took his bequest and their talks to heart, and nearly twenty years later she established the first modern hospice.

In her long career—she was still seeing patients at St. Christopher's in London at age 82—Saunders was a nurse, a social worker, a physician, and a pharmacology researcher. Her multifaceted perspective on terminal illness gave rise to the concept of "total pain," a complex web of physical, emotional, social, and spiritual elements that she felt was best addressed by an interdisciplinary team. After working as a nurse at St. Thomas's, where patients with all sorts of conditions were thrown together in a large, chaotic ward, and then as a social worker at St. Luke's, where the dying received somewhat better treatment, she realized just how much better care of the dying could be. A surgeon with whom she worked encouraged her to go into medicine, telling her, "It's the doctors who desert the dying, and there's so much to be learned about pain. You'll be frustrated if you don't do it properly."[30] With the psychological backing of her mentor and the financial backing of her father, she started medical school at the age of 33.

After completing a research fellowship in pharmacology that allowed her to systematically study approaches to pain relief, and after ten years of applying her knowledge to the care of patients at the St. Joseph's Irish Sisters of Charity hospital, Cicely Saunders was ready to launch her own hospice. From its inception, St. Christopher's embodied all the features of today's hospices: a focus on home care, a recognition that care of the dying is a family matter, and a systematic approach to bereavement. She also incorporated research and teaching into her model program. Today, St. Christopher's has 500 home care patients, a 40-bed inpatient unit, a substantial staff, and a slew of volunteers.

Thanks to Cicely Saunders, care of the dying has become a recognized discipline in its own right. It draws on the expertise of psychiatrists, social workers, chaplains, and other nontraditional caregivers to achieve the goal of dying well.[31] In principle, there is no reason why we cannot develop good hospice care for dying patients while simultaneously allowing physician-aided death. In fact, there is some evidence that in Oregon, legalizing PAS served as a spur to improving end-of-life care. Suddenly aware that patients might actually kill themselves if their pain was not well managed, hospitals and physician groups took seriously the need to do a better job of caring for dying patients. When palliative measures were instituted in patients who had requested PAS, nearly half decided not to proceed with suicide.[32] In practice, PAS is intended as a solution to the problem of dying poorly, not as a stimulus to hospice referrals. But the secret to dying well is not to turn death into the ultimate opportunity for self-determination. Rather, the key is the assurance that your friends, your family, and your physicians will care for you and keep you comfortable until the very end.

FOUR

The Trouble with Medicare

Most americans believe that once you turn 65, you will have to worry neither about getting health care nor about paying for it. You will be entitled to Medicare, the national health insurance program enacted into law in 1965, which you think will cover all your needs.[1] The one widely acknowledged flaw in the program, the lack of a prescription drug benefit, was remedied by the Medicare Modernization Act of 2003.[2] With this new addition, it seems like a perfect program. In fact, Medicare does not cover a great many beneficial treatments and services, ranging from eyeglasses and hearing aids to long-term nursing home care. The net effect is that elderly people today are paying more out of pocket for health care than they did before Medicare was introduced.[3] But the problem with Medicare is not just what it leaves out of its package of "covered services." A deeper, more intractable problem is that embedded in the Medicare program are powerful incentives that shape the kinds of decisions that physicians, hospitals, and patients make—and these incentives serve to *dis-*

courage them from using exactly the kinds of treatment that make sense for huge numbers of older people, such as intermediate and palliative care.

Medicare *is* an excellent program—for the most vigorous of older people. It is no surprise that Medicare serves very robust elders well, since it was originally designed to provide coverage for older patients with episodic, reversible disease. It works beautifully for a person with an acute illness such as a kidney infection or gallstones, which typically requires a brief hospital stay and a short course of treatment—antibiotics for the former and surgery for the latter.

But if Medicare is a good program for robust elders, it is profoundly inadequate for people who are frail or who are nearing the end of life. The reason for this inadequacy is that it favors institutional care over home care, it supports technology-intensive treatment rather than labor-intensive care, and it fails to provide adequately for chronic diseases.[4] And people who have multiple medical conditions or are near the end of life fare best with care that keeps them out of hospitals, that helps them manage chronic illness, and that substitutes low-technology treatment for invasive therapy.

MARTIN BLACK was one of my many frail patients. He was 89 years old and had severe diabetes that sent his blood sugar levels ricocheting from very low to sky-high over the course of a single day. His diabetes had affected his vision, so he depended on his wife to draw up insulin in a syringe and to give him the injections. He also relied on her to test his blood sugar several times a day. Actually, Martin depended on his wife for a great many other things as well—his memory was not what it had been in the days when he was a successful accountant who remembered the names of all his clients and all their family members and was up on every government regulation pertaining to taxes. Martin had never mastered household tasks—he had always left the cooking, shopping, and cleaning to his wife, and he decided that he was not about to take on any of those chores after he retired. In fact, apart from balancing the checkbook, which had been his job since their marriage sixty years ago, all the other household tasks fell to his wife, Minnie.

Martin was known for his sharply creased wool slacks, pressed button-down shirts, and gleaming leather shoes. The trousers and shirts were always solid-colored, as befitted a respectable older man—most often navy below the waist and white above. It was only his ties that were outré. One year he had sported tiny pigs with the caption "MCP"; another year he wore a tie covered with whiskey bottles. Most people thought that he was the fashion-conscious one and never suspected that Minnie selected his clothes and chose the ties. Without her, he was helpless.

If Martin was dependent on his wife to get by, he was also at the mercy of his assorted medical conditions. The slightest perturbation plunged him into a cascade of medical catastrophes. Just before his ninetieth birthday, when his wife was helping him put on his trademark designer slacks, she noticed that his left leg was swollen. Always on the lookout for skin problems—he was prone to infections because of his diabetes—Minnie immediately took him to the local hospital emergency room. To her surprise, the doctor did not think he had an infection, but rather another common medical condition, deep vein thrombosis (DVT), or a blood clot in the leg. This is a potentially serious problem: if untreated, the blood clot can travel from the leg to the lungs, where it is renamed a pulmonary embolism. Clots in the blood vessels of the lungs can wreak havoc, producing shortness of breath and even death.

The Blacks were told that the treatment for DVT was hospitalization and administration of an intravenous blood thinner. However, they were not informed that there is a newer treatment that involves two injections a day of a different but related type of blood thinner. The older approach, using the drug heparin, requires frequent blood tests to determine whether the patient is receiving the right amount of medication. Too much heparin is dangerous—it can cause bleeding from the intestines, bleeding into the brain, or bleeding at other undesirable locations; too little heparin means a risk of further blood clots. The newer approach, using a modified form of heparin, is considerably simpler. The dose of the medication is determined by the patient's weight, and no monitoring of blood tests is required. What is even more remarkable is that preliminary outcomes of treatment using the newer, easier method are actually better than the outcomes with the old treatment.[5]

From the patient's point of view, the shots make more sense than a continuous infusion. Surely it is far better to stay at home and receive two injections each day than to enter the hospital. At home, Martin would be cared for by his doting and vigilant wife, who would know exactly what food he would eat and what he wouldn't. She would detect immediately if he was not himself, a potential sign of low blood sugar. But the standard treatment for DVT when Martin developed his blood clot was hospitalization, and that is what Medicare would pay for. So Martin was admitted to a medical ward. Disoriented, he repeatedly got out of bed and promptly fell in the unfamiliar, poorly lit room. His doctors felt they had no choice but to sedate him with medication. He stopped trying to get up but in his restlessness pulled out his intravenous line. The doctors decided to tie down his arms. Martin was confined to bed for the next five days, which left him weak and wobbly.

From the vantage point of cost, home care has to be cheaper than hospital care. It's true that the new type of heparin is pricier than traditional heparin, and since most patients do not know how to give themselves an injection, a nurse would have to come to the home twice a day to give the injection. But the cost of the medication and the visiting nurse is far less than the cost of even a few days in the hospital. The average national payment by Medicare for treatment of DVT in the hospital—exclusive of physician visits—is $3,400. Even with overpriced pharmaceuticals and the inefficiency and hence relatively high cost of home nursing care, the home alternative is significantly cheaper.[6]

Despite the clear cost advantage of home over hospital care, Medicare pays for heparin and nursing care in the hospital—no questions asked—but might not pay anything at all for treatment at home. Although medications are covered for outpatients as of 2006, they are not included if the patient's total annual drug costs are between $2250 and $5100. Martin Black, who took insulin for his diabetes as well as assorted other medications, would easily run up an annual bill of $3000 for his regular medications, which means he would fall right into the "hole" created by the Medicare Prescription Drug Law.[7] And Medicare would pay for a nurse to administer the shots at home only if his doctor certified he was "homebound."

To enable Martin to be treated at home, the harried emergency room physician would have had to make all the necessary arrangements. She would have had to make sure a nurse was available to administer the shots (not always easy, particularly on weekends and holidays). She would have had to find a pharmacy that stocked the special heparin—again, not always an easy task if the drug is not routinely used at home and therefore is not commonly stocked by local pharmacies. Instead, the doctor told Mrs. Black that her husband needed to be admitted to the hospital. The hospital was set up to handle his sort of problem, and Medicare is structured to pay the hospital to take care of it. The fact that home care makes both human and medical sense—and in this case economic sense—was beside the point.

Medicare also shows that it favors high-tech solutions to medical problems by encouraging hospital care for a variety of conditions that could be adequately treated in the less technologically-intensive environment of the nursing home. When Martin Black developed pneumonia, just two months after he recovered from the blood clot in his leg, and needed round-the-clock nursing care, oxygen, and perhaps intravenous fluids, he could in principle have received that care in a skilled nursing facility. But Medicare regulations require that in order to be eligible for admission to a nursing home, a patient must stay overnight in a hospital for three days, so Martin went back to the hospital, where he again became confused and was sedated and restrained.

If the three-day rule simply meant that Medicare favored an expensive option (hospital care) over a less expensive alternative (skilled nursing facility care), it would be regrettable but not hazardous to health. In fact, not only is hospitalization costly, but it is also risky. In Martin's case, hospitalization left him profoundly weak and debilitated. He was therefore transferred to a nursing facility for rehabilitation before returning home. Over the course of his illness, he went from his physician's office to the hospital emergency room, from there to a general medical floor, and then on to a nursing home. The multiple moves characteristic of a modern-day hospital stay are frequently disruptive and potentially dangerous.[8] Every time a patient transfers from one setting to another, a physician has to transcribe his orders. Each time the medication orders are rewritten by the physician at the receiving end of the transfer, a process that is currently done by hand, there is a chance of an error. When patients move from one site to another, their new caregivers often do not know anything about their baseline status. They cannot judge what medical problems are new and which ones are old. As a result, patients such as Martin who develop acute confusion—a state which is both serious and treatable—are often mistakenly thought to have dementia, and patients who are depressed—which is likewise serious and treatable—are often misdiagnosed as being withdrawn or cognitively impaired.

Gone are the days when patients remain in the hospital until they are well enough to go home. Before the advent of diagnosis-related groups in 1983, a system in which Medicare reimburses a fixed amount for a given diagnosis, regardless of the length of stay, patients were typically cared for in the hospital by the same doctor who had cared for them before their admission and who would continue to follow them after discharge. Today, driven by Medicare's reimbursement policies, hospitals are eager to discharge patients as soon as possible. The hospital, after all, is paid the same amount for a patient with a hip fracture regardless of whether he stays for two days or ten (the rate is based on the expected stay of five days), but costs rise with length of stay. As a result, short-term skilled nursing facilities have proliferated to provide care for patients who are no longer sick enough to justify a hospital stay but who are not well enough to return home.

Medicare, in its eagerness to promote efficiency and decrease costs, was the impetus for the current fragmented system of care. Its reimbursement strategies shaved off days at the end of a hospitalization and substituted skilled nursing facility care for those days. Paradoxically, however, its focus on technologically-intensive medicine has not allowed consideration of an alternative strategy, direct admission to a skilled nursing facility, which could both promote efficiency and avoid potentially hazardous transfers. What people with frailty so desperately need, and what is missing from conventional Medicare, is care that offers continuity, coordination, and comprehensiveness. Martin Black was hospitalized for treatment of the blood clot in his leg in part because there was no one to arrange all the services that would have been required for him to stay at home. He needed a case manager to make sure a nurse came to the house twice a day and that he had the medication and the needles and syringes to administer it. He needed a doctor willing to go to the Blacks' home to check whether his leg was getting better. For a physician to be able to measure improvement, the same physician had to evaluate him in the office, the emergency room, and his home—or at the very least, Mr. Black needed a team of doctors and nurse practitioners who communicated seamlessly with one another.

The team is essential because maintaining the health of a frail older person is as dependent on social workers, physical therapists, chaplains, and nurses as it is on physicians. The importance of a team has been shown over and over again—in geriatrics, in palliative care, in addressing the problems of chronically ill children and of patients with AIDS. Typical teams are composed of a physician, a social worker, and a nurse, who serve as the core and who call in other members as needed. A member of the team has to be available any time of the day or night, since emergencies occur at all hours. Night is the most perilous time because family members often panic at night, and frail, sick people who show up in an emergency room at 2:00 A.M. are almost certain to be admitted to the hospital even if they would be better off with home care.

Martin Black would have benefited from integrated care at the level of the people who provided the services; such coordination is most easily achieved if there is coordination at the level of the organizations that pay for those services. If the same insurer or health plan is financially liable for care regardless of whether it is administered in the intensive care unit or the home or the nursing home, it is in that organization's interest to ensure that there are no barriers to the preferred form of care. It would be in the best interests of both Martin Black and his health insurance company to treat his pneumonia in a skilled nursing facility, not in a hospital. He needed managed-care Medicare that truly managed the care of complex patients with multiple needs.[9] Such a program would be willing to invest in an interdisciplinary team because it would not be bound by a fee-for-service mentality: social workers and nurse practitioners who engaged in counseling would be paid, with the recognition that the benefit of their work might only be realized months later, when the advance planning process resulted in a choice of medical over surgical treatment.

The area of end-of-life care illustrates all of Medicare's perverse incentives—use of high-tech rather than low-tech care, substitution of institutional care for home care, and a focus on acute rather than chronic illness. Many terminally ill patients are hospitalized for management of symptoms such as pain, nausea, or shortness of breath. These patients will typically receive aggressive treatments and diagnostic tests, rather than exclusively palliative care; one study of patients with advanced dementia or metastatic cancer found that 49 percent received one or more nonpalliative treatments during their terminal hospitalization.[10] Likewise, Medicare favors hospital care over home care for terminally ill patients, with the exception of those enrolled in hospice, because home care, like skilled nursing facility care, is difficult to arrange without a prior hospital stay. As a result, 50 percent of people over 65 die in the hospital and only 25 percent at home, although the vast majority would prefer to die at home.[11]

Even the hospice program, in which patients can enroll if they have a prognosis of less than six months, though very well-regarded by participants and their families,[12] focuses primarily on the actively dying patient. However, end-of-life care should also be seen as treatment for patients with a "serious and complex illness," a condition that is disabling, progressive, and ultimately fatal.[13] That hospice care is widely viewed by patients and physicians alike as care for the dying is reflected in the fact that the median survival of patients after enrollment in Medicare hospice programs is 16 days, and 25 percent of patients die within 7 days.[14] While an exclusive focus on comfort care makes sense for many patients whose death is imminent, a combination of palliative and curative treatment may be quite reasonable for patients whose prognosis is less certain or who are not psychologically ready to accept the label of "terminal illness." The current reality is that the majority of patients who are near the end of life receive technologically-intensive care in a hospital and enroll in hospice, if at all, only when they will die in a matter of days or weeks. Restructuring the incentives within Medicare would allow patients with a serious and complex illness to be eligible for home care without denying them the possibility of hospital treatment.

Older people who are near the end of life are ill-served by Medicare. With its powerful incentives to provide nursing home care rather than home care and curative rather than palliative treatment, Medicare undermines the goal of comfort. The result is needless suffering as well as a high price tag.

MARJORIE SAMSON was a saint in that all too rare sense of having performed an arduous and often thankless task with supreme competence and good cheer. At the age of 55, just when her four children had all become self-sufficient, Marjorie found herself the caregiver for her parents, both of whom, in an unusual twist of fate, had Alzheimer's disease. For a while, they took care of each other: Allan's memory was not as far gone as his wife Joan's, so between the two of them, they could figure out how to microwave precooked meals and run the dishwasher. They devoted themselves completely to household tasks, with the result that most of what needed to get done was accomplished. Some days, Joan mopped the kitchen floor three times while the bathrooms languished, accumulating the unmistakable smell of urine. Allan and Joan always bought a quart of milk when they went to the grocery store, so depending on how many other items they needed over the course of a week, their refrigerator could be stocked with as many as ten quarts of milk. When Marjorie discovered they had made two mortgage payments in one week but hadn't paid their credit card bill in months, incurring the typical usurious fees, she took over their finances. When she found out they had ruined three saucepans by leaving them on the stove long after the last molecule of liquid had been vaporized, she arranged for home-delivered meals. And when she realized that they had given up bathing after an episode in which the tub overflowed, flooding their entire apartment, she decided to move them to her own house and take care of them.

For five years, Marjorie provided personal care for Joan and Allan Englund. She did the shopping, the cooking, and the house-cleaning. She took them to medical appointments and the barber, and she paid their bills. Allan spent most of his days in a recliner because he had a bad knee. Joan had nothing wrong with any part of her body except her brain. Her only coherent words were "thank you." She responded to her name and seemed to regard her husband and daughter as vaguely familiar, but she never called them by name. Marjorie quit her part-time job as an accountant to spend more time with her parents. She continued to whistle while she worked. But when she strained her back helping her father out of the bathtub, her long-suffering husband insisted that something had to change.

Handing over the entire care of her parents to strangers was out of the question for Marjorie. She did not believe that anyone else would change her mother's diapers or dress her father with as much patience and affection as she did, and she was probably right. But Marjorie was a realist, so she hired aides to do the heavy care, supervising them closely, and continued with the less back-breaking work herself. Over time, her parents needed more and more help, and much of the work was physical. Allan could no longer get out of a chair unassisted—and he was a husky man who had never lost his linebacker physique. In contrast, Joan was an elf—barely five feet tall, skinny, with her hair still brown at age 80. From behind, she could be mistaken for a scrawny pre-adolescent. She was agile and it was easy enough to lift her legs or arms when dressing her, but she was in constant motion and liable to get into mischief if she didn't have a spotter at all times.

Too tired to chase her mother all day, and no longer able to provide personal care to her father, Marjorie asked about Medicare home services. She discovered that from Medicare's perspective, her parents were too healthy to qualify for a homemaker to do chores or a home health aide to provide personal care. They were not even, strictly speaking, homebound—another prerequisite for Medicare services.[15] They certainly couldn't go anywhere on their own—Allan had been the driver in the family, and he had given up driving years earlier. Their sense of direction was far too unreliable for them to go on a bus by themselves. But Joan could get into someone else's car without any difficulty and Allan could be maneuvered into the back seat, although it took some doing.

Then Allan fell and broke his hip, after which he was eligible for home services for a few weeks. But then he became "too stable," and he no longer qualified. The assistance evaporated. Marjorie dipped deeper and deeper into her parents' savings to hire helpers. When the money was gone, they went on Medicaid, the joint federal/state program providing health care for the poor. Once they were on Medicaid, they could enter a nursing home and virtually the entire cost would be borne by the state. Although Medicare does not pay for long-term nursing home care, Medicaid does. In fact, most nursing home care is paid for by Medicaid, with a small portion covered by the Veterans Administration (for qualifying veterans), a tiny bit by long-term-care insurance, and the remainder paid for privately.[16]

From the perspective of the Medicare program, institutional care for frail elders is domiciliary care: it involves room and board. Medicare is a medical program, not a social or housing program. But for older people who are unable to take care of themselves because of overwhelming physical disabilities—such as those that arise from a stroke or Parkinson's disease, or a combination of problems such as heart disease plus severe arthritis, or significant cognitive impairment (usually from Alzheimer's disease or another form of dementia)—the distinction between the physical and the social is blurred. Medicaid, which provides health care for the poor, is also a medical program but it *does* pay for nursing home care. Thus, there is a financial incentive for frail older individuals to receive their care in a nursing home rather than at home. If Medicare paid for nursing home care, there would be no such incentive; but as long as there is an opportunity to "cost shift," institutional care makes more sense than home care.

Almost no one prefers nursing home care to remaining at home. Some older people have claimed they would rather die than go to a nursing home.[17] While their view often changes when they are faced with an actual rather than a theoretical situation, and while their views may reflect outdated notions of what nursing homes are like, there is no question that staying home is the preferred alternative. Going to a nursing home may not really be a reason to commit suicide, but that doesn't mean it is a desirable option.

The economics of home versus nursing home are less clear. There are certainly economies of scale associated with institutional care: one aide can take care of six, eight, or even ten nursing home residents, depending on their degree of disability. Similarly, one nurse can provide care to upwards of fifteen people—in some instances as many as forty people if they principally need help with personal care rather than with medical monitoring. On the other hand, nursing homes do not separate room and board from medical care—they provide comprehensive care (although some components are usually omitted from coverage, such as clothing, visits to the hairdresser, and telephone service). The average cost of one year of care in a nursing home is $61,685, with Medicaid reimbursement rates varying markedly depending on the location.[18] That translates into a great many hours of home care, whether for a nurse (typical hourly rate of $49) or a home health aide (average hourly rate of $28) or a homemaker (usual hourly rate of $18).[19] Clearly, an individual requiring round-the-clock care could easily spend over $61,000 per year. But the person who needs someone to come in four hours a day to help with washing and dressing, and perhaps someone to come in eight hours a week to cook and clean, and then a nurse to check her blood pressure once a month, would cost the government a great deal less than $61,000 each year. On balance, many—though by no means all—of the frail older people who currently enter nursing homes might be able to remain at home if Medicare provided an incentive to keep them there.

With great reluctance, Marjorie arranged for her parents to be admitted to a local nursing home. They shared a room and she visited daily, but it was still vastly inferior to their setup in her house. Confused as her mother had been at home, she became noticeably more so in the nursing home. She no longer said "thank you," she smeared toothpaste on her clothes, and she tried to eat a bar of soap.

Within a few months of her admission, Joan stopped eating soap, but she also stopped eating her meals. A tray with multiple dishes was overwhelming to her, so the staff put one plate in front of her at a time. But she had increasing difficulty figuring out what to do with the utensils—sometimes she tried to eat her soup with a knife or her chicken with a spoon. Finally, the nurses concluded that she should be fed and put her at a table with three other "feeders," assigning an aide to spoon-feed the entire group. That approach worked for a while, but Joan tended to become distracted while eating; she found watching her companions more interesting than chewing, which took considerable effort. Sometimes she stopped chewing her food, and sometimes she neglected to swallow it. Mealtimes expanded until it took an hour for Joan to eat half the food on her plate. She began losing weight, and the nurses worried that the nursing home would be branded "deficient" by state regulators because Joan Englund was malnourished. They strongly recommended to Marjorie that she allow them to send Joan to the hospital to have a gastrostomy tube inserted.

Marjorie did not want her mother to have a feeding tube. She did not think her mother would want one either, or would not have wanted it had she been able to understand her predicament. But the nursing home was adamant—they would not spend an hour three times a day spooning food into a reluctant resident. The Medicare program gives nursing homes a financial incentive to switch from the labor-intensive, time-consuming process of feeding patients with the help of aides to the use of tube feeding. If a long-term resident of a nursing home has a feeding tube inserted, she may qualify for transfer to a "skilled nursing facility." This is often just a different bed in the same nursing home, where her care will be reimbursed at a higher rate simply because she has a new feeding tube. After several weeks, she will be moved back to the chronic rather than the acute part of the nursing home. But even in the chronic section of the facility, reimbursement rates in much of the country are higher for patients who have a feeding tube in place, although the cost of hand feeding is less than that of tube feeding.[20] The staff told Marjorie that she could feed her mother herself or hire a private aide to feed her. If she did not or could not provide additional help, the facility would be happy to arrange for hospitalization for the procedure—or for transfer to another nursing home.

Marjorie felt she had no choice: she agreed to the placement of a feeding tube. Three months later, still malnourished and suffering from pneumonia, Joan Englund died. Two months after that, Allan died in his sleep at the nursing home. The diagnosis on her father's death certificate was Parkinson's disease, but Marjorie thought that a broken heart would have been more accurate.

If medicare is deeply dysfunctional for frail elders and for those approaching the end of life, how should it be reformed? The key is that the one-size-fits-all model does not work for older people, who are a heterogeneous group with vastly differing needs that depend not on their chronological age but on their overall state of health. The Medicare program has implicitly acknowledged this reality by creating two distinct alternatives to conventional Medicare for a fairly small segment of the eligible population: the Program of All-Inclusive Care of the Elderly (PACE) for the frail and the hospice program for the terminally ill. The criteria for enrolling in these Medicare variants are so restrictive that not many have done so (in the case of PACE), and those who do join (in the case of hospice), are only in the program for a very short period: PACE has only 10,500 members nationwide, and the median length of hospice enrollment is 16 days.[21] The overwhelming majority of older people continue to subscribe to traditional Medicare, whether the fee-for-service or the capitated variety. But these alternative versions of Medicare, suitably modified, can form the basis for a new system of three discrete packages offering an intensive, a comprehensive, and a palliative approach to care.

The intensive package would look similar to the current Medicare program. It would be targeted to robust older people, who in general have fared well with the current Medicare services. A few crucial ingredients are missing from contemporary Medicare: complete coverage for eyeglasses, hearing aids, dentures, and prescription drugs. These will have to be added to the Medicare mix if vigorous older people are to remain robust as long as possible and not lapse into frailty because their poor vision leads them to miss a step, fall, and break a hip. It may be necessary to use means testing to determine the premium for the additional items. In addition, Medicare has been slow to provide preventive services, and some of the screening tests it does cover are generally inappropriate for the older population: it omits hearing screens, which have been shown to be effective, and covers prostate specific antigen (PSA) testing, which has not. The current program has been expanding, with osteoporosis screening, glaucoma testing, mammography, and influenza vaccination recently added to the list of covered services. Those changes for which there is good data should be covered in the new intensive version of Medicare.

The comprehensive package, suitable for older people with multiple chronic diseases, would build on the PACE model. PACE originated with the On Lok Senior Health Services program in the 1970s. Designed to serve the Chinese-American community, it was based on the assumption that frail older people didn't want to enter nursing homes but needed a lot of support to stay out of them. The key component of the On Lok program was the adult day health center, where its members congregated during the day and received various services including podiatry, nursing, and physical therapy. On Lok was a social as well as a medical program: its founders recognized that in order for it to work, the staff would need to provide transportation, emotional support, advance planning, and all sorts of other services that were not routinely discussed, let alone offered, by medically oriented programs. It was also a capitated program, supported by joint Medicare and Medicaid funding.

The On Lok project was so successful that the federal government, together with the Robert Wood Johnson Foundation, decided to support several other demonstration projects created on this model. Programs were launched in nine sites across the country. As a result of their ability to simultaneously improve the quality of care and to decrease costs, an unbeatable and rare combination, the federal government in 1997 switched PACE from "demonstration" status to "permanent provider" status. As of 2005, thirty-two PACE sites were serving 10,500 patients.[22]

What PACE does is to connect patients with an interdisciplinary team, consisting at a minimum of a physician, a nurse practitioner, and a social worker. Other professionals such as physical therapists and dieticians, as well as drivers and home health aides, are called in as needed. The team members assess patients, develop a plan of care, and address acute problems when they arise. Since these problems can occur at any time of day or night, and holidays and weekends are not exempt, a system is in place to provide hands-on care 24 hours a day, seven days a week. PACE team members are familiar and comfortable with advance planning. They recognize the need for patients' involvement in their own care and for family support to cope with chronic illness. Remarkably, PACE doesn't prohibit hospitalization or restrict ICU care. It does such a good job of caring for patients at home that the use of aggressive and invasive care is far lower than with conventional Medicare.

To make this program a realistic option for the millions of elderly people with multiple chronic diseases, and not just the handful who use it today, we will need a new version. This new package will get rid of the requirement for dual Medicare and Medicaid eligibility, which has limited PACE to low-income patients. The insistence that patients must be nursing home–eligible will also have to go. Right now, 63 percent of Medicare patients have at least two chronic diseases, and 20 percent have at least five chronic conditions. All of the latter and many of the former could benefit from a comprehensive Medicare package, but most of them aren't ready for a nursing home.[23] In addition, the services now offered at adult day care centers such as podiatry and dentistry would need to be arranged by a case manager, and the program would need to provide transportation for patients to see those providers. For the program to gain wide acceptability, the adult day health center could no longer be the central locus of care.

The comprehensive package would have to pay for a number of interventions that promote independence, such as hearing aids, glasses, and dentures. For the program to be fiscally sound, a few deletions from the current Medicare menu would be necessary, principally invasive technological interventions that offer little chance of prolonging life and a significant risk of impairing its quality.[24] An example of a technology that would not make sense for elderly patients with multiple chronic conditions is the recently approved left ventricular assist device—essentially an artificial heart chamber implanted in the abdomen. This device is used in patients whose heart disease is so severe that they would be candidates for a heart transplant if they did not have so many other chronic diseases. Although these pumps prolong life to a greater extent than does medical therapy, half the recipients are dead within a year and many are plagued by bleeding and infections during the extra months they gain.[25] Other comparably invasive technologies would likewise be excluded, such as lung volume reduction surgery, an operation used in patients with certain forms of advanced emphysema that involves cutting out the most badly damaged parts of the lungs. This expensive surgery does not even prolong life—its goal is to improve exercise tolerance and decrease shortness of breath.[26] But in a frail person, the side effects of a major surgical procedure like this are likely to outweigh any symptomatic benefit.

The third alternative, the palliative package, would build on the hospice program. Hospice, like PACE, centers on a team approach to care. It is holistic, attending to psychosocial and spiritual issues as well as to symptoms and diseases. It does not include hospital care but instead seeks to ensure that patients get what they need at home. However, it limits participation to people with a prognosis of six months or less and excludes coverage of life-prolonging treatment. The new Medicare benefit would be designed to focus on comfort—not to the exclusion of life-prolonging treatment, but incorporating such care only if it doesn't produce major discomfort. The package would offer ample home services so that, unlike the situation today, patients could enroll in hospice even if they did not have family members to provide essentially full-time care. It would include hospital care—if it is necessary for comfort. It would explicitly cover chemotherapy and radiation treatments if their overriding goal is to maintain comfort, regardless of whether, as a side effect, they happen to prolong life. This represents a departure from current hospice programs, which do not cover curative therapy for the underlying fatal disease. Because treatments such as radiotherapy, which is typically given five days a week for several weeks, are both expensive and may be interpreted as curative, many contemporary hospices choose not to offer them. Hospice programs are paid a fixed daily rate, regardless of how much they spend, so they clearly have an incentive to avoid very costly treatment. What is now hospice would be expanded to include patients with terminal conditions such as advanced dementia or end-stage heart failure. These patients often fail to meet the current eligibility criteria for hospice care—the requirement that they have a prognosis of six months or less. This criterion makes good sense for most cancer patients, who can be reasonably free of symptoms and quite functional until they fairly abruptly reach a turning point in their illness. It makes far less sense for patients who have a progressive, ultimately fatal illness other than cancer; their course is far more likely to involve a stepwise deterioration or a gradual dwindling rather than a precipitous decline.[27]

Offering three discrete benefit packages would be no more complicated than the current options available to the Medicare population: today, on reaching age 65, a prospective patient can select conventional Medicare or Medicare Advantage (formerly called Medicare plus Choice).[28] If the individual chooses traditional Medicare, he has to decide whether to purchase Medicare Part B, which pays for physician services and laboratory tests and comes with an extra premium. Next, the patient has to decide whether to purchase Medicare Part D, the voluntary prescription drug benefit. Finally, he must decide whether to supplement Medicare with a "MediGap" policy that provides additional coverage for items not covered by regular Medicare, such as co-payments and deductibles.

Alternatively, the patient can select one of the Medicare Advantage plans available in his area—principally health maintenance organizations (HMOs) that have contracted with the federal government to provide capitated care. These plans, like HMOs in general, have the advantage of simplicity—you show your card and, after a co-payment for office visits and medication, you receive service. In fee-for-service Medicare, by contrast, you receive complicated bills in which you are charged a deductible and then 20 percent of Medicare's allowable rate for the service, a rate that may bear little resemblance to the fee charged by the physician. If the physician "accepts assignment," then his actual charge is meaningless; the government sets the rate. In states where the physician does not need to accept assignment, the patient may be billed for a portion of the difference between what Medicare covers and what the physician charges.

Deciding which HMO to opt for is also complicated because each has different co-payments and different covered services (for example, some include glasses and hearing aids; others do not). Because their formularies differ, HMO plans offer varying medication coverage. Moreover, the managed care plans charge an additional premium (on top of Medicare Part B, which enrollees also have to pay) in exchange for the extra services.

The three plans—intensive, comprehensive, and palliative—have the virtue of being conceptually distinguishable. Older patients would choose which plan made sense for them based on their understanding of their underlying health condition and their personal goals of care. Of course, for people to be able to make reasonable choices, they have to know what their condition is, which means their doctors have to tell them. Physicians are notoriously poor at discussing prognosis, particularly when patients have multiple diseases and their overall prognosis reflects the combined effects of those conditions.[29] If physicians learn to discuss health status and prognosis frankly with patients, most patients will make choices based on their status. The majority of robust people will select the intensive plan, most frail people will opt for the comprehensive plan, and the majority of dying patients will select the palliative plan, once they understand whether they are robust, frail, or near the end of life. Offering patients choices is the preferred route, but if, after a trial period of offering the various benefit packages, few people choose anything other than conventional Medicare, we should consider assigning benefits on the basis of health status.

This idea is not as radical as it sounds. There is nothing discriminatory about offering different kinds of treatment to people with varying conditions, any more than it is discriminatory to treat "pneumonia" differently depending on whether the patient has AIDS, dementia, or sickle cell disease as well. Patients with AIDS are at risk for *Pneumocystis carinii* pneumonia, an otherwise rare form of pulmonary illness; patients with dementia are at risk of aspiration pneumonia (essentially, they inhale bacteria that normally live harmlessly in the mouth); and patients with sickle cell disease are at particular risk of pneumococcal disease. Each of these kinds of pneumonia requires its own diagnostic tests and treatments. Treating all three types identically, out of a misguided sense of egalitarianism, would be harmful to all these groups of patients.[30]

We routinely accept the notion that where we work determines what health care benefit package we receive. Employees who work for a particular company are eligible exclusively for the health insurance plan offered by that company, with whatever restrictions the plan provides. If we change jobs, we may well have to change health insurance coverage and participate in a different plan with a distinct set of benefits. We also regard as perfectly acceptable the idea that age can determine health care coverage: once a person turns 65, he typically loses his insurance coverage and becomes eligible, instead, for Medicare, which may not have the same provisions as his previous insurance. We are comfortable with the current approach of using economic status as a basis for determining insurance benefits: poor people are eligible for Medicaid, which offers different coverage from private health insurance plans. And finally, we are evidently satisfied to allow place of residence to determine benefits: health insurance plans, including Medicaid, vary markedly in terms of their coverage from state to state. It is actually much fairer to determine what health care benefits you receive on the basis of your *medical* needs rather than your job, your age, your income, or what state you live in. Elderly patients are heterogeneous: those who are robust benefit from episodic, acute care; those who are frail due to multiple chronic illnesses benefit from coordinated, long-term care; those who are near the end of life benefit from a palliative approach.

The main difficulties with such a system would be figuring out who gets which benefit package and when it's time to switch to a different package. At first glance, limiting a given treatment in some circumstances but not others seems hopelessly complicated. However, many health insurance plans currently make different coverage decisions depending on the specific clinical circumstances. The Medicare program, for example, will reimburse for plastic surgery to correct a malformation created by oncological surgery or arising from trauma, but would deny coverage for an analogous procedure that was requested on purely cosmetic grounds. Most insurance plans will cover a bone marrow transplant for acute leukemia, a condition for which it has been shown to be effective, but will not pay for a transplant in a patient with breast cancer, a condition for which it has not. The recent decisions to cover the left ventricular assist device and lung volume reduction surgery are restricted to patients meeting particular clinical criteria.

The challenge in the case of invasive, expensive treatments for elderly patients is to determine fairly and justly who is in fact frail and who is nearing the end of life, and then to conclude which treatments are reasonable. Underlying health status could be assessed in outpatient geriatric assessment clinics or at the time of hospitalization, using criteria that reflect disease severity, functional status, and cognition.[31] Testing Medicare recipients to determine which benefit package they should receive, while alien to current thinking, could become as routine as an eye examination for the renewal of a driver's license. The examinations would need to be repeated periodically to identify changes in health status.

Since its inception, the Medicare program has only covered services that are "medically necessary," but there is no uniformly accepted definition of medical necessity. The language of the original Medicare legislation indicated that "no payment may be made . . . for any expenses incurred for items or services . . . which are not reasonable and necessary for the diagnosis or treatment of illness or injury or to improve the function of a malformed body member."[32] Most authorities interpret this to mean that services are medically necessary if they "meet the standards of good medical practice."[33] Medicare has consistently opted to exclude from coverage many effective medical procedures that it regards as inappropriate: for example, it will not pay for laser treatment of nearsightedness. There is no reason why Medicare should not choose what treatments to cover in the treatment of frail elders or dying elders on the basis of their appropriateness.

Reconfiguring Medicare will not occur overnight. We need to begin by establishing just what the standard of care is for conditions such as advanced dementia or extreme frailty. The best way to do that is with a consensus conference under the auspices of the National Institutes of Health that would bring together all interested parties, including physicians, social workers, nurses, clergy, and the lay public. While such consensus conferences have typically focused on the optimal treatment of specific diseases such as osteoporosis or incontinence, others have addressed certain types of patient, such as the pediatric patient or the maternity patient. An example of a model consensus process was the town meetings held in Oregon to prioritize coverage decisions for the state's Medicaid program. By inviting representatives from the health care professions, community groups, religious groups, and others, the Oregon meetings managed to balance efficacy of treatment, impact of the disease on individuals and society, and cost. We need to initiate a similar process at the national level, with separate task forces considering the right mix of health care for elderly people who are robust, those who are frail, and those who are dying. Once there is agreement on both general principles and the details, we can begin the challenging task of translating the plan into reality.

FIVE

Is a Nursing Home in Your Future?

THE LATEST prediction is that if you are just now turning 65, you have nearly a 50 percent chance of spending some time in a nursing home before you die. Approximately 10 percent of these nursing home stays will be short-term, intended for recuperation after a hospitalization.[1] The remainder will be for the long haul, with discharge to a funeral parlor, not to the family home.

Just how many baby boomers will live permanently in a nursing home in the future depends on developments in health care and housing and on the rate of disability in the coming years. The best estimates are that the numbers of residents will climb from 1.6 million in 2003 to somewhere between a low of 2.6 million and a high of 5 million in 2050.[2] Whichever estimate turns out to be correct, we will need substantially more long-term institutional care than we have now as the baby boomers reach old age. In large measure, the reason is the anticipated growth in the number of people over age 85. The growth in demand for nursing home care will also arise from the fact that while overall disability rates have declined—they fell about 1 percent per year between 1982 and 1999—there has been no decline in the fraction of older people with *extensive* disabilities, the people most likely to need institutional care rather than assisted living or home care.[3] In addition, the diseases that make people dependent in their old age are not vanishing or even diminishing. If anything, arthritis, Alzheimer's disease, and visual and hearing problems are on the rise.[4] If the baby boomers want to be certain of being able to find a good nursing home, in the event that we need one, the time to begin working on changing the nursing home industry is now.

For years, Paul Dimaggio had volunteered at his local nursing home in his spare time. He had helped transport wheelchair-bound residents to activities and appointments within the sprawling, multi-level facility, and for a brief period he had led a Veterans Reminiscence Group. Sharing World War II stories was good for the residents, some of whom had experienced the camaraderie and the intensity of army existence as the high point of their lives, but it had been hard on Paul. He had been a prisoner of war, and all the stories brought back memories that gave him nightmares. He also found it exasperating that no one ever seemed to speak loudly enough for all the others to hear, which meant he was constantly trying to summarize what each person said, tersely but forcefully. There were residents who took the floor and monopolized the discussion, recounting their history in excruciating detail, often telling the same story every week. Some of the participants were tolerant of the repetition, but others complained vociferously. Paul didn't like the bickering and he found the repetition tedious, so he gave up the group and stuck with providing transportation. Now, although he was having trouble processing the new reality, he was being admitted to the nursing home himself.

The first stop was the financial office. For the third time—Paul had already had a screening evaluation and a pre-admission visit —he had to prove he was who he said he was. He had to show his birth certificate and his Social Security card. Then he had to ver- ify that he had medical insurance coverage, handing over his Medicare card to be photocopied. Most important, he had to demonstrate that he was one of the dwindling numbers of older people who have sufficient personal resources to pay for nursing home care out of pocket. Paul presented his bank statements and his investment portfolio report and signed an affidavit allowing the nursing home to deduct his room and board directly from his bank account, a stunning $9800 per month. The national average for semi-private nursing home care is $61,685 per year, or just over $5100 each month, but this was a superior nursing home in an expensive part of the country.[5]

The second stop was the floor where he would be living. For expediency, he was escorted to his room in a wheelchair, probably one of the same heavy, basic models he had pushed around as re- cently as the previous year. Accompanied by his son, Rudy, who repeatedly brushed a stubborn lock of hair out of his eyes, Paul was shown his new room by the nursing home's social worker.

It was a long, narrow room, almost entirely filled by two paral- lel beds, with a nondescript, shabby curtain suspended between them. "This is your bed," the social worker told Paul, pointing toward the entrance, the side furthest from the window. The walls were beige and looked as if they were due for a new coat of paint. The floor was linoleum—smooth, washable, and reminiscent of a high school classroom. The room boasted a single closet, divided in half for each of its occupants, and a bathroom with a sink and toilet. Next to the bed was a night table; along the remaining free wall was a small bureau and, above it, a few shelves for books or photographs or personal knickknacks. A vinyl-covered chair was wedged in between the door and the bureau. Until this morning, Paul had lived in the three-bedroom colonial where he had brought up his two sons, a home he had shared with his wife of 60 years until her death six months earlier. All he had taken with him were two suitcases of clothes, a photo album, framed pictures of his wedding day and his sons' college graduations, a clock radio, and a calendar. Everything else, 88 years of accumulated memories, had been given away, thrown away, or in a few cases, stored with his sons.

Paul looked at the room, one that was identical to so many rooms to which he had delivered residents in the past. It had the same standard-issue bed, bureau, and bookcase. The decor did not vary—once-white window curtains that looked gray no matter how often they were washed, and a pale green bedspread that reminded Paul of the complexion of his fellows soldiers during his troopship's trans-Atlantic voyage. He thought fleetingly of his own furniture—the leather recliner that had been his present to himself on his 80th birthday, the soft living room sofa with the plump cushions that he had had reupholstered for his 50th wedding anniversary. His regrets, if that's what he was experiencing, were interrupted by the arrival of his roommate.

Charlie was a big man who used a rolling walker. "You like to watch the ballgame?" he asked by way of introduction. "I turn in every night at eight except when there's a game on. As long as you don't snore too loud, we'll get along fine." He shuffled into the bathroom and slid the door shut in a vain attempt to keep his excretory exertions private.

That evening, Paul discovered that he could no longer take his medications when he chose. The nurse on duty dispensed his regular medications at the time designated by his new physician, whom he had not yet met (or the approximate time, since one nurse distributed medications to thirty nursing home residents). At eleven P.M., when he still had not fallen asleep, Paul rang for the nurse and requested a sleeping pill: at home he had regularly taken medicine against anxiety, and when he had difficulty sleeping, he popped an extra tablet. At the nursing home, he was told there was "no order" for a sleeping pill, or for any anti-anxiety medicine, and was given a Tylenol tablet instead. Paul did not think Tylenol was likely to help him—he didn't have a headache or any other kind of pain, and moreover he had never found Tylenol useful even when he did have pain, but the nurse assured him it worked like a charm for many of the residents.

He finally dozed off around midnight, woke up several times during the night when the nurse came by to pat him down, which was her way of checking for incontinence, and entered a deep sleep just as the sun began to rise. He got his next taste of nursing home life when a cheery nursing assistant woke him at seven A.M., determined to get him up and dressed. Paul insisted that he didn't need anyone to get him up, he could dress himself, and in any event, he wasn't ready to get up. The nursing assistant was friendly but firm. She had just one hour to get eight residents dressed and into the dining room to await the arrival of the breakfast trays. They could not all wake up at five minutes to eight. He was the new kid on the block—those with the greatest seniority had the most desirable wake-up times. And, she added, sizing Paul up as a troublemaker, skipping breakfast was not allowed.

Paul had moved into a relatively good nursing home, with competent staff and enough of them, at least according to federal standards.[6] But his new "home" was very different from his own home—it was an institution, all-encompassing, bureaucratic, and structured to keep its residents safe and clean and organized for the convenience of the staff.

Mental hospitals, orphanages, boys' prep schools, convents and, some would add, nursing homes, have been labeled "total institutions."[7] They have much in common: they all have entry rituals in which they effectively strip members of their previous identity and redefine them by a particular feature such as their medical history (or crime committed). All the activities of their occupants—eating, sleeping, and bathing—take place in the same location; there is never an escape to a more neutral locale. Total institutions make inmates dependent on staff members, who have almost complete authority over their every move, and they restrict access to the outside world. To put it simply, a total institution is organized to promote efficiency among the staff rather than to meet the specific, individual, and variable needs or wishes of its residents. It is typically dedicated to a single overriding goal—serving God in the case of a convent, and the health and safety of residents in the case of a nursing home.[8]

Paul Dimaggio quickly learned to hate the nursing home to which he had previously been so devoted. Moving in, signing forms, divulging personal information, and allowing the nursing home direct access to his bank account—all of these he experienced as pure submission. He felt much the way he had when he gave his consent for a surgical procedure, except that had been a one-time event and he'd been asleep during the operation. The move to a nursing home would almost certainly be the last stop on life's journey, and it was a stop during which, Paul realized, he would remain exquisitely awake and aware.

The nurses were capable and compassionate, if a bit harried. Paul particularly liked the nurse on duty from three to eleven P.M., who often sat with him for a while when he couldn't sleep or when he was anxious and afraid. "I'm no good for anything," he would tell her. "I wish I were dead," and then: "I don't want to die." The nurse tried to distract him. She listened to stories of the pharmacy he had owned for many years, until the third break-in by thieves in search of narcotics persuaded him it was too dangerous a business. The aides, who helped Paul get washed and dressed, were a mixed bunch. One Jamaican woman who worked on weekends was extraordinarily gentle. She checked whether he was ready before starting to dress him; she asked him to lift his arms instead of ordering him around, or worse, moving them for him as though he were a doll. Some of the other nursing assistants were rough and their tone was harsh, hassled, impatient. But Paul learned quickly that he was dependent on the staff for everything. They could come promptly when he asked for help going to the bathroom, saving him from the excruciating embarrassment of what was euphemistically known throughout the nursing home as "an accident." They could make sure they changed the bandage on his leg ulcer early enough to allow him to leave the home on a trip to hear a Boston Symphony Orchestra rehearsal— or they could sabotage his escape by repeated delays. Apart from an occasional trip and the periodic lunch date with his son, who lived nearby, Paul spent his entire day on his "nursing unit." He ate with the same group of forty residents three times a day, he watched movies with them, and, if his interests had been in that direction, he would have played bingo with them.

What made Paul distraught was not just the power the staff exerted over him, though he found that irritating, especially when the wielders of power were short-tempered nursing assistants. Nor was it his sense of confinement, though he yearned to have the physical stamina to go on walks outdoors by himself. What bothered him was his overwhelming feeling of uselessness. He was accustomed to helping others: as a neighborhood pharmacist, he had given customers advice about pain-killers, about treatments for hemorrhoids and diarrhea, about contraception. When he retired, he had volunteered in the nursing home in order to do something tangible for the less fortunate. Now he was one of the less fortunate, and he saw himself as completely superannuated.

A recreation therapist came to see Paul to discuss what he liked to do—what kind of music he liked, whether he might enjoy playing cards. But Paul was not interested in entertainment—it was too passive and too fundamentally self-centered. What he wanted was *work*. And that, except for some rare opportunities to stuff envelopes or distribute napkins, was unavailable in the nursing home.

Many nursing home residents, unlike Paul Dimaggio, are happy to be entertained and want to be taken care of. But even residents who wish to be served want things done their way— they want to exercise a modicum of control over their lives. The essence of most nursing homes, by contrast, is that residents cede all except the most trivial decision-making authority (they are routinely asked what they want to wear). Giving up control might not be a problem if the nursing home and the resident shared the same goals. But the predominant goal of most nursing homes is the safety of its occupants, whereas the overriding goal of those occupants is typically to enhance their quality of life, even when this entails taking risks with safety. For many nursing home residents, the freedom to walk independently, without waiting for a nurse escort, is more important than minimizing their chance of falling, despite the associated risk of breaking a bone. Other nursing home residents would prefer to sleep through the night undisturbed rather than being awakened every few hours to check the bedclothes for evidence of incontinence, even if lying on damp sheets predisposes them to skin breakdown.[9]

To design a nursing home where frail older people can thrive, we have to start by asking about the residents' goals—not about the families' priorities and expectations, which is what the sales and marketing experts pay attention to. Middle-class families, who are usually the ones doing the looking when it's time to find a nursing home for mom, are impressed by the public spaces: the lobby, the café for visitors. They tend to imagine that a good nursing home resembles a hotel with plenty of amenities. But hotels are for transients, temporary residents who typically are out most of the day and who use their room as a base of operations rather than a place to live. And of course hotels are not set up for people who are incontinent and cannot dress themselves.

Individuals who live in nursing homes, at least those who are sufficiently cognitively intact to articulate their concerns, say that what's important to them is to be able to decide when they get up and when they go to bed, who their roommate is (or better yet, not to have one), and what they eat. They want to be able to make phone calls, to get in touch with their own physicians, and to go on trips outside the nursing home.[10] They want those things that they regard as essential to maintaining their quality of life—and if quality conflicts with safety, they would opt for quality. Most nurses and aides who work in nursing homes, however, think that residents care primarily about organized "activities" such as bingo, arts and crafts, and movies.

Not all nursing homes are as resolutely convinced as was Paul Dimaggio's facility that they know what is best for their residents. Beginning in the early 1990s, reports coming out of one nursing home, Providence Mount Saint Vincent in Seattle, suggested that something special was happening there. The Mount, as its occupants call it, was said to be a good place to live, not just a place to wait to die.[11]

The leadership of Mount Saint Vincent, which was originally a conventional nursing home, decided in 1990 to give the facility a philosophical as well as a physical overhaul. They recognized that older people can overcome apathy and dependence if they feel valued as individuals who are part of a community. To be respected as persons means maintaining some degree of control over their own lives, and to be considered members of a group means physical stability—in the case of living in a nursing home, remaining in the same room. The new Mount, which took ten years to create, is divided into small neighborhoods in which residents "age in place." Instead of moving from one floor to another as they developed increasing degrees of impairment, with the top floor always the "worst" place to be, occupants joined a wing of the facility and stayed there until their death. Nursing assistants were empowered to design their own schedules in partnership with the people for whom they provided care. The residents, in turn, had choices in the areas of life that mattered to them. By all accounts—and none of the accounts take the form of objective social science research—the Mount has made significant progress in nurturing relationships and facilitating meaningful activity.[12]

Providence Mount Saint Vincent is part of a movement aimed at creating cultural change in nursing homes. A handful of organizations committed to nursing homes that focus on the quality of life of their residents have banded together under the banner of the Pioneer Network.[13] Their precepts are straightforward: the nursing home should revolve around the needs and wishes of its residents, and that means attending to spiritual as well as mental and physical concerns. The Pioneer Movement also recognizes both that the experience of the residents is critically dependent on their relationships with staff, particularly nursing assistants, and that nursing homes have a history of devaluing and exploiting their nursing assistants by providing inadequate training, paying minimal wages, and giving them little control over their work lives. The Pioneer movement, at least in principle, values both residents and staff as unique individuals, people who can make a difference in the lives of others.

THE PIONEER MODEL is not the only version of cultural change in today's nursing homes. The Eden Alternative is another strategy that aims to banish boredom and loneliness—in this model, by introducing animals and plants into nursing homes. The movement was founded by Bill Thomas, a Harvard Medical School graduate who did his residency at the University of Rochester, home of the biopsychosocial model of medicine.[14] As he describes his own personal journey, Dr. Thomas says he became burned out from the endless torrent of disasters that were the mainstays of his work. As he put it: "I took a job as a physician at a nursing home . . . because I thought that it would be a break from my real work as a[n] ER doctor. And I fell in love with the work. And I fell in love with the people. And I came to detest the environment in which that care was being provided."[15] He concluded that the ennui and growing dependency he observed in nursing homes were a result of residents' isolation from the larger community. Working with his wife Judy, Bill Thomas decided to make the walls of the nursing home permeable to the outside by including pets (dogs, cats, birds, and rabbits are the most common), plants, and children in the lives of the residents. Founded in 1991, about the same time that Providence Mount Saint Vincent was remaking itself, the Eden Alternative shares many features with other cultural change movements. One of its cardinal tenets is that when staff members are well treated by an organization, they will in turn treat the elders in their care well: nursing homes must be good places in which to live *and* to work. Another core principle is that teamwork is superior to a hierarchical, bureaucratic structure for getting things done, and that it is far more conducive to good relationships between staff members and elders. The flora and fauna that populate Eden buildings are symbols of the deep commitment to making these homes a place where life abounds.

Bill Thomas's newest venture is still another variation on the theme of cultural change. Known as the Green House model, this plan involves six or eight frail older people living in a house with round-the-clock care. More akin to a group home than to a conventional nursing home, the idea grew out of Thomas's personal experience. He and his wife Judy learned that their older daughter, then a newborn, was afflicted with Otahara's syndrome, an extremely rare neurological condition. The child had severe seizures; she was blind; she could not walk, sit, or even raise her head unassisted. Two years later, their second child was born with the same condition. The Thomases decided to keep their daughters at home, with a staff of ten caregivers providing 24-hour care. The parents coordinate all the social services and medical care that their children require. It's exhausting, but it works, and as Thomas said in an interview explaining how he came up with the Green House concept: "We don't care for our girls with a housekeeping department and a nursing department . . . everybody participates to get the girls what they need."[16]

Despite extraordinary efforts on the part of the leaders of the cultural change movement, the number of facilities that endorse its principles remains small, and their work is largely unknown to the general public. Only 300 out of 16,400 nursing homes have an Eden certificate, indicating that staff members have attended Eden training sessions and that at least some of the Eden principles have been introduced. Although the Pioneer group has held its own conventions and attended national meetings of professional organizations to spread its message, only a dozen or so homes today are thoroughly resident-centered.[17] Little formal research has been done to test whether resident-centered care results in greater happiness, better health, and less depression. If families are going to vote with their feet by refusing to admit an elder to a conventional nursing home, they have to know the facts and what to demand, but in most communities there are no models of what institutional care really can be. There are a few hotbeds of change, including Seattle and Rochester, where the new ideas have caught on and seem to be contagious. Once a facility opens up that embodies cultural change, other nursing homes in the area are apt to modify their structure, perhaps because of the publicity surrounding the novel institution and the opportunity to see one in action. But outside the few pockets of progress, and apart from a scattering of stellar nursing homes whose leadership intuitively treats each resident with respect and dignity, most of the country is a nursing home wasteland. One of the most powerful means of counteracting the prevailing tendency is information. Information about nursing home quality is increasingly available to consumers, but regrettably, it glosses over the most critical determinants of quality.

W HEN NANCY FARRELL reluctantly decided that her mother needed to live in a nursing home, she consulted the government Web site called "Nursing Home Compare."[18] She wanted objective information on which to base the decision about where her mother should go, which is exactly what the site provides. For every American nursing home that is Medicare- or Medicaid-certified, this Web site provides four pieces of information: demographics (size and profit or not-for-profit status); performance on a set of "quality measures"; the number of deficiencies identified at the last state inspection; and staffing ratios. Comparisons are presented with state and national averages. Nancy looked mainly at the quality measures. She did not pay much attention to what they were actually measuring, but trusted that they were a good reflection of the overall quality of care at the facilities. Armed with the information she got from Nursing Home Compare, Nancy visited two nursing homes near the insurance company office where she worked. She liked the idea that she could drop in during her lunch hour or on her way home or even before the beginning of the work day, sampling different shifts of nurses and nurse's aides in the process. She also consulted the federal government's guide to choosing a nursing home. She selected the newer of the two places she visited, which had a sunny lobby with lots of plants, and where no resident was still in bed after eight A.M. One month later, her mother moved into a sparsely furnished double room at the Emerald Gate Nursing Home.[19]

Edna Farrell was petite, opinionated, and 87 years old. She had suffered a mild stroke, she had moderately advanced Parkinson's disease, and in case that wasn't enough to profoundly limit her mobility, she also had severe arthritis affecting her hips and knees. Nancy was delighted when the facility recommended a physical therapy consultation for her mother. But Edna took one look at the therapist, a bouncy young woman in running shoes who sported a pin saying "Yes you can," and announced: "I don't want to walk."

The therapist tried coming at different times of day. She asked Edna whether her joints hurt when she moved. "No, I'm just tired," was the answer. The therapist suggested checking Edna's blood count—perhaps she was tired because she was anemic. But Edna was not anemic, nor did she have an underactive thyroid gland or an undiagnosed urinary tract infection, any of which, in principle, could sap her energy. Maybe, her daughter theorized, Edna was depressed. She had always been sociable and had enjoyed attending lectures and concerts. Now, Edna said, going out required too much effort. She wanted to be left alone. I didn't think Edna was depressed: she had a good appetite, she slept well, and she did not feel worthless or unfulfilled. She was content to sit in her room, into which she had managed to squeeze a small writing table, and write letters to old friends or sort through old photographs or read best-sellers. "As long as I can still read, I'll be okay," she told me. "I don't have the energy to go places or do things. I'm comfortable in my room with my children and my grandchildren around me"—she meant the pictures on her book-shelves—"and with my favorite sweater handy if I need it." In an expansive moment, she elaborated further: "I've traveled to lots of countries. It was all very interesting, but the truth is that traveling is a monumental pain. And now they make you take your shoes off at the airport. Do you know how difficult it is for me, with my stroke and my arthritis, to take my shoes off? And if I say I can't, they get suspicious." With that, Edna waved me off, making it clear that she would likewise dismiss the physical therapist and the psychiatrist and whoever else tried to "motivate" her.

Edna entered Emerald Gate using a walker, and within six months she needed a wheelchair to get around. She gave up eating in the nursing home's central dining room because leaving the floor where she lived was too difficult. From the perspective of the quality measures used by Nursing Home Compare, Emerald Gate had failed with Edna. It had allowed a woman to deteriorate—and she had not even broken a hip or suffered a heart attack as an excuse. The nursing home had merely acceded, albeit grudgingly, to Edna's wishes.

To many people like Edna, regaining or even maintaining their mobility is simply not important. That doesn't mean the nursing home should not have offered Edna physical therapy. It doesn't mean the nursing home does not need to have physical therapists readily available, preferably on staff, to work with residents who are interested in their services. But the overriding goal of the nursing home should be to promote quality of life. For some individuals, quality of life is closely bound up with mobility, and restoring their ability to get around on their own is crucial to their life satisfaction. For Edna, however, walking was a chore—an anxiety-laden, physically burdensome chore. She worried that she would fall. She was so slow that walking wasn't an efficient means of getting to her destination. It hurt to walk. She was far happier learning to use a wheelchair—and probably would have experienced even greater freedom had she been able to zip around in an electric wheelchair. Maintaining mobility in the nursing home should be the means to an end, not an end in itself. By accepting "the percentage of residents who decline in their daily function" as a measure of institutional quality, the federal government encourages nursing homes to adopt maximization of function as its major objective.[20]

The immutable reality is that almost all long-term nursing home residents develop greater disability over time. Occasionally, someone enters a nursing home who is over-medicated or who is just beginning to recover from a serious illness and who, with a little ongoing physical therapy and a lot of encouragement, makes great progress. By examining the rate of decline, the government hopes to distinguish between facilities that neglect their residents, leaving them to sit for hours in the hallway, bored and immobile, and those that stimulate their residents, encouraging them to walk and to participate in various activities. In the extreme, this differentiation is useful. I would not want my family members or my patients in a nursing home where all they did was to vegetate. But to expect that everyone who is not explicitly dying will maintain whatever level of independence he had on admission is at best naive and at worst dangerous.

Nursing Home Compare will tell you about other markers for

poor care, such as infection rates and restraint use. These are moderately useful measures.[21] I would certainly prefer to be in a facility that recognizes that tying people down is an attack on their dignity and does not even have the desired effect of protecting them from falling. A facility that continues to use a lot of restraints, despite the federal law restricting their use that went into effect in 1987 and despite the adverse publicity associated with them, is probably benighted in other ways as well. The use of restraints is a likely indication of other kinds of unfortunate attitudes and behaviors on the part of staff and administrators.

Several months after her admission to Emerald Gate, Edna Farrell fell out of her wheelchair. She was in severe pain and her right leg was rotated to the side, as typically happens when a person has broken her hip. I arranged for her transfer to the local hospital emergency room. It was a wintry day when everyone in Boston seemed to have developed pneumonia or a heart attack or to have fallen on the ice. There were no beds in the hospital, and there would not be any until a few fortunate patients were discharged. As a result, Edna waited on a stretcher for fourteen hours before she was finally transferred to a bed in a conventional hospital room. As it turned out, she had broken her hip and had been unable to shift her weight as she lay on the stretcher. She was totally dependent on the harried emergency department staff to move her from side to side. Because of her hip pain, she received sizable doses of morphine, and as a result she did not experience the normal restlessness that most people feel when they are in the same position for a prolonged period. She had not even wiggled around when she was lying on the stretcher.

After Edna underwent surgical repair of her broken hip, her nurse noticed that she had a gaping wound on her buttock— the side opposite the hip fracture—an opening that extended through the outer layer of skin and into the tissue deep underneath the skin. Lying motionless in the emergency room for all those hours had led her to develop a pressure ulcer or bedsore. When Emerald Gate heard about the pressure sore, the administrator suggested transferring Edna to a different facility, one that specialized in wound care. At first, her daughter Nancy liked the idea of a nursing home with experts in pressure sores for her mother. But the more she thought about it, the more disturbed she became. Edna had finally adjusted to the original home, and the staff had gotten used to her. They were no longer badgering her to walk, and they knew there was no point getting her up for breakfast because she didn't eat breakfast. And the recommended special facility was twenty miles from Nancy's office instead of within walking distance. She decided to ask just how important a transfer would be for her mother's recovery. What she learned was that the original nursing home had its own wound care nurse specialist and used the same low-pressure mattresses and special dressings as the other facility did. The difference, as far as she could tell, was that if Edna went back to Emerald Gate, she would show up on the facility's roster of patients who had developed pressure ulcers. Pressure ulcer rates constitute another quality measure, and Edna Farrell would be a black mark on the nursing home's record if she returned from the hospital with a sore that was unlikely to heal completely in the next three months.[22] Nancy Farrell put her foot down: her mother was going to go back to the place she had come to consider home.

Once she returned to Emerald Gate, a new battle began. Edna didn't have much of an appetite, and she didn't drink a lot of fluids. The pain medication she took before each dressing change dulled her appetite as well as her pain. Without it, she was in agony. With it, she didn't eat much. The nurses decided that the best way to monitor her for dehydration was to weigh her every day. However, Edna could not stand on a scale. The attendants tried weighing her on a special chair scale, but that approach still required transferring her from the bed to a chair. She could not stand unassisted, and although she only weighed 125 pounds, she was dead weight. One of the nurse's aides injured her back so badly when trying to maneuver Edna that she was out on disability for six months. To move Edna from the bed to a chair, the staff began using a lift, a contraption which cranked her up into the air and then propelled her from one place to another. Edna was terrified of the lift. She was convinced the staff would drop her. She was frightened that the aides would be called away while she was suspended in midair and would leave her hanging. She worried that the straps that held her would break. Edna didn't cry or scream when she was in the lift, but she whimpered like a hurt animal.

The purpose of weighing Edna every day was to monitor her for evidence of dehydration and malnutrition, since she was eating poorly and drinking erratically. The majority of older people lose the exquisitely sensitive thirst monitor that makes starvation or being stranded in the desert so terribly uncomfortable for younger individuals. Between Edna's abnormal thirst mechanism and the diuretics she took for her blood pressure, she was at risk for dehydration. Dehydration, in turn, can cause confusion, weakness, dizziness, falls, and even death. The rationale for monitoring for dehydration is to intervene before severe symptoms develop. As soon as a resident's weight drops a pound or two, the physician can put the diuretic pills on hold, order the nurses to ply her with fluids and, if the weight loss is five pounds rather than merely two, insert an intravenous line to tank her up.

But did Edna want such assiduous attention to her fluid status? She hated all the poking and prodding she had been subjected to in the hospital. She dreaded the twice-daily dressing changes for her pressure ulcer. The lift gave her nightmares. Edna wanted to be comfortable; surely she would not want her life to revolve around fending off dehydration. In the extreme, if she became profoundly dehydrated she would be too lethargic to tool around in her wheelchair and could even die—a fate she indicated, in her darker moments, she would welcome. Considering the cost to Edna of all the weighing and the blood tests, wouldn't it make more sense just to develop a heightened recognition that if she got a fever, for instance, she would need extra fluid and probably should stop taking her diuretics temporarily?

The motivation behind all the monitoring was a desire by Emerald Gate to take good care of the vulnerable old people in the facility's care. It was also a desire to avoid a citation for inadequate care when the state surveyors came around. Nursing home administrators live in fear of the surveyors, who are supposed to visit, unannounced, on average once a year. They do not visit substandard nursing homes more often nor superior ones less often—they are required by law to show up yearly and look for "deficiencies." Each nursing home gets a report card after its survey, which is publicly available. In many states, it is posted on the Internet. Nursing facilities proudly advertise themselves in local newspapers as being "deficiency-free," which is a little like a mother boasting that her award-winning high school senior is a "non-C student." If the facility racks up enough bad marks on its scorecard, it receives "sanctions," which range from small fines to larger fines to being closed down.

The state surveyors interpret and enforce federal regulations, of which there are an extraordinary number. Some have claimed that the only industry that is more tightly regulated in America than nursing homes is the nuclear power industry.[23] The rules are codified in the Code of Federal Regulations, which despite the blandness of its name and the tedium of its contents is the book that determines the everyday aspects of life for nursing home residents. The rules even specify the temperature at which meals must be served—which is the reason residents have to be seated in the dining room, awaiting the arrival of the meal trays from the kitchen like runners at the starting line, ready to spring into action at the sound of the starting gun. The rules also dictate that nursing assistants must receive a specified amount of training, which has been interpreted to mean that friendly volunteers, who have not had the requisite training, cannot do things such as escort residents to the bathroom.

The National Nursing Home Reform Coalition, the major advocacy organization for nursing home residents, went to tremendous lengths to make sure that the regulations focus on outcomes and that they have teeth. This represents progress—nursing homes are no longer supposed to be evaluated on the basis of their notebook of policies and procedures, but rather on whether they do what they claim they do. And if they don't, they are penalized. This revolutionary change went into effect with the Omnibus Reconciliation Act of 1987, widely called OBRA and also referred to as the Nursing Home Reform Act. Powerful as this legislation has been in cleaning up nursing homes where residents were routinely tied in their seats, sedated to keep them quiet, and left to develop pressure ulcers after sitting motionless in urine-soaked diapers, it has also indelibly stamped nursing homes as *institutions* devoted to health and safety.

Shortly after the passage of OBRA, well-intended researchers created a new instrument to comprehensively assess the health and physical functioning of all nursing home residents.[24] Unfortunately, it ensures that nursing home staff will measure and record the activities of residents instead of interacting with them and responding to their needs. Every certified nursing home in the country must complete this "Minimum Data Set" (MDS) on each resident annually, with shorter quarterly updates and extensive re-evaluations whenever there is a "change of status," which is jargon for getting sick.[25] It is from the MDS that surveyors would learn that Edna Farrell was at risk of dehydration and malnutrition. They would then check to make sure that Emerald Gate was taking the appropriate steps to protect her. As long as she was weighed daily and had blood drawn periodically, the surveyors would be satisfied. If the facility heeded her piteous cries to be left alone, it could be cited for inadequate care.

Thanks to federal intervention, nursing homes have evolved from fire traps warehousing the elderly into medical institutions with recommended staffing ratios, strict sanitation codes, and mandated nutritional standards. The price for these improvements has been the re-creation of the nursing home in the image of the hospital. Government regulation, though historically responsible for the elimination of the most florid abuses in nursing homes, has consistently focused on health and safety rather than quality of life.[26] Even the typical physical layout of the nursing home mirrors the conventional hospital, with its long corridors, shared bedrooms, and central nursing station, which is the hub of activity. The residents are regarded as patients whose "activities" are regimented. Bingo, current events, and of course meals are scheduled at fixed times for an entire cohort of elders. The purpose of the institution is ostensibly treatment of medical conditions: hence games are not "entertainment" but rather "recreation therapy," and music and art are not pursued for their own sake but instead packaged as "creative arts therapy."

Today's nursing homes are run by professional nurses, dedicated to restoring and maintaining health, even though more than 60 percent of the care required by residents is *personal* care —help with dressing, bathing, or using the toilet. And the personal care itself is provided by nursing aides who work under the supervision of nurses rather than by attendants whose focus is on companionship and social interaction. Physicians, to the extent that they are a presence at all in nursing homes, tend to be satisfied with the institutional view of the nursing home. It has traditionally been inconvenient for physicians to travel to nursing homes to see patients, and as a result few of them continue to take care of their patients once they enter a nursing home. Those who do travel to nursing homes to see patients spend, on average, less than two hours per week providing care in this setting.[27] Much of medical practice for nursing home residents is conducted by telephone or in hospital emergency rooms, to which acutely ill residents are sent with alarming frequency.

Studies of the quality of care in nursing homes before and after the introduction of the Minimum Data Set suggest that overall quality has improved. What is not clear is whether the improvement is actually due to the assessment process or to other simultaneous changes, such as more or better staff, or slightly greater physician involvement in nursing home care. It should also be noted that the studies purporting to show better outcomes were conducted by the same researchers who created the MDS in the first place.[28]

How can we hope to create the kind of nursing homes we could actually imagine living in if the regulatory model pushes us to build institutions that are safer, cleaner, and ever more impervious to the messy business of emotions and relationships that give meaning to old age? The answer is not to abolish regulations. Unfortunately, professionals cannot be relied upon to police themselves; we have ample evidence of the need for external monitoring from the annals of medicine and nursing. Nor can nursing home administrators be relied upon to do the right thing for the vulnerable incapacitated elders in their charge, especially though not exclusively in the for-profit chains. The first critical step toward radical new models of nursing home care is greater public awareness. The vast majority of Americans don't realize how problematic long-term care is in the United States, and almost assuredly do not know what determines quality in nursing homes. Polls continue to show that 74 percent of people mistakenly believe that Medicare will cover long-term nursing home care after age 65.[29] They may be vaguely aware of abuse and neglect in nursing homes, since these issues were widely publicized by muckraking books such as *Tender Loving Greed* and *Unloving Care: The Nursing Home Tragedy* in the 1970s,[30] but they are also generally aware that the quality of care has improved in recent years.

If we want cultural change to revolutionize nursing homes, we will need a major shift in the focus of government regulation. For it is the regulations, promulgated at the federal level by the Centers for Medicare and Medicaid Services (CMS) and implemented at the state level by departments of public health, that drive the organization of nursing homes. The regulations will need to change in a very simple way, simple in theory if not in practice: they will need to shift from quality of care (defined as health and safety) to quality of life. At some level, CMS recognizes that this approach makes sense. After all, the most surefire way to keep old people free of injury, such as lacerations and hip fractures, would be to sedate them into oblivion, tie them down, and feed them through a tube. Of course, this ultimate form of safety would come at a price—the ability to interact with the world. Leaving aside whether a person who is comatose or nearly so can be thought of as disease-free (surely medication-induced coma itself is a disease, albeit iatrogenic), ignoring for a moment that restraining and sedating someone itself predisposes that person to skin breakdown and pneumonia, obviously the point of maximizing safety is to facilitate life, not to squelch it.

Social scientists at the University of Minnesota have recognized how critical it is to be able to define and measure quality of life in the nursing home. They have come up with eleven discrete domains to capture quality, ranging from relationships to meaningful activities—something other than bopping balloons, a prototypical nursing home recreational activity. A sense of safety is another domain, but feeling secure is very different from being free of injuries. In a similar vein, a sense of privacy is a domain, which is measured not by whether everyone has a private room, but by whether residents can easily find solitude if they want it. Autonomy and freedom of choice is a domain—to the extent that the individual is interested in making choices and able to do so. Some of the domains have to do with how people in a nursing home are treated, regardless of what they experience: individuality, for instance, has more to do with staff members knowing and respecting a person for who he has been and what he was like, whether or not he can still express his identity.[31] The Minnesota group has been successful in attracting the government's attention and has received a contract to develop a short, reliable instrument for assessing quality of life in American nursing homes based on the eleven domains.

If the Centers for Medicare and Medicaid Services are going to bother with a new and philosophically very different instrument, the baby boomers will have to exert direct pressure. The federal government has invested a huge amount of money in the Minimum Data Set, which does not measure quality of life and does not pretend to, although it pays lip service to caring for the whole person. The government will need truly compelling reasons to jettison an established tool for a new one.[32] The best way to exert that pressure is to build a vibrant consumer movement. Bill Thomas, founder of the Eden alternative, says that the baby boomers won't stand for conventional nursing homes and will insist on something better: "The baby boomer generation is coming. And the irresistible force of the baby boomers is about to collide with the unmovable object of the nursing home. And there's going to be an explosive charge that comes from this collision."[33] But if the boomers wait until we are old and sick, we won't have the energy to demand change. If on top of being old and sick we are demented, we won't come close to having the capacity to demand much of anything. The time to act is now.

In addition to developing incentives to create the kinds of nursing homes where we can imagine living, we will need to figure out ways to bolster the long-term-care labor force. We can come up with innovative models of resident-centered care for nursing homes, but if we don't have the manpower—or in this case, more accurately, the womanpower—to provide the care, all the regulations and safeguards and imagination will not lead to successful implementation. Unless we take steps now, we are facing a labor shortage of gargantuan proportions.

To put it simply, the number of people who will need direct care will more than double between now and 2050. Conservative estimates suggest that the number of elderly individuals using either nursing facilities, assisted living, or home care services will go from 8 million today to about 19 million in 2050.[34] At the same time, the traditional supply of both paid and informal care-givers will be shrinking. Informal caregivers—who provide about three-quarters of all care, and whose services have been valued at $196 billion—are primarily spouses and adult children. But couples are having fewer children—some are having no children—and the divorce rate is rising, all of which decreases the supply of potential informal caregivers. Paid caregivers—the paraprofessionals who provide the vast majority of care in nursing homes and at home—are typically between the ages of 25 and 54 and are overwhelmingly female. The certified nursing assistants in nursing homes are 90 percent female; home health aides employed by agencies are 96 percent female; and all self-employed home health aides are women. As educational opportunities increase for poor women, especially minority women, the pool of potential paraprofessionals can be expected to decrease.

To meet the projected needs of the elderly, the number of long-term-care workers will need to grow at a rate of 2 percent per year from now until 2050, in a period when the working-age population overall is growing at a rate of only 0.3 percent per year.[35] It's not just the necessary percentage increase that is staggering; it's the absolute numbers. One fairly conservative estimate is that the number of long-term-care workers needed, all told, will go from 1.9 million today to 4 million in 2050. Shifts of the elderly population from nursing home to assisted living to home won't matter—disabled elders will need personal care wherever they are. In fact, more helpers will be necessary if a larger fraction of the care is given at home, since the ratio of caregivers to old people is usually 1:1 in the home (perhaps 1:2 if both members of the couple need assistance) rather than 1:6 or 1:8 in the nursing home. Declines in disability rates among the elderly won't help the situation because the decreases to date have been in the need for help with things such as cooking, shopping, and housekeeping, not in the need for help with bathing, dressing, and walking—precisely the problems for which older individuals use personal assistants. Technology may improve matters slightly: for example, computerized reminder systems could help residents in assisted living remember to go to the dining room for meals, and microwave ovens and online grocery shopping have already helped older people retain their independence. But we aren't going to be able to rely on robots to give an octogenarian a bath or get him dressed. Many disabled elders can put on their own shoes thanks to Velcro straps and long shoe horns, but they have to be able to distinguish the right shoe from the left and to know that their socks go on first and then their shoes. People with dementia, the largest subgroup of those who will need long-term care in the future, will have to rely on human assistance to get by.

The possible solutions to the labor shortage problem are reasonably straightforward, if only we have the will to implement them. To attract more workers into the field, wages and benefits have to improve. Currently, the national average hourly wage for an aide in a nursing home is $8.29, compared to $9.22 for a service worker. Only 76 percent of aides hired by nursing homes and only 68 percent of those employed by home health agencies have health insurance.[36] To retain employees, the job has to become more attractive. That means more respect, more autonomy, and fewer injuries for workers, as well as prospects for advancement.

Today, home health aides, certified nursing assistants, and personal care attendants are at the bottom of the employment barrel. They have one of the highest injury rates of any industry: in 1999, 13 out of every 100 employees lost work time as a result of injury, compared to 8 out of 100 in construction.[37] Innovations that give paraprofessionals more control over their jobs, more flexibility, and greater respect, such as those instituted by a coalition of Midwestern nursing homes called Wellsprings, have successfully increased job satisfaction rates and decreased turnover—which is often as high as 100 percent a year in nursing homes. But even these significant improvements were not sufficient to actually increase the numbers of people interested in becoming nursing aides. Several states have created career tracks within nursing that enable women to start out as aides and advance to become a licensed practical nurse. This strategy has yielded important but modest increases in the numbers of women entering the field.

Perhaps a more promising strategy is to try to squeeze more help out of family members, although they already provide 70 percent of all caregiving to older people. If families received a moderate amount of financial support, a guarantee of periodic respite, and information about supplementary services, maybe they could do more. The National Family Caregiver Support Program provides some degree of help, primarily in the form of information about available services, but proposals to legislate a tax credit (of up to $3,000 a year) have been defeated under both Presidents Clinton and Bush. Each of these approaches—and we need to use all of them—costs money.

The single most effective means of increasing the labor force has been to put more money into long-term care. Strategies to address the labor shortage cannot be left to individual nursing homes or entrepreneurs because they require systemic changes in education and enhanced long-term-care financing, which is now principally derived from Medicaid. As taxpayers, we are going to have to acknowledge that if we want to ensure an adequate supply of caregivers in the future, we're going to have to spend more, not less.

All of these measures may, in the end, still be insufficient. A job that requires minimal training (even if it carries with it the possibility of promotion), and that is inherently physically and emotionally stressful, may simply be unappealing to most Americans, as long as they have other alternatives. We may have no choice but to increase the number of caregivers through immigration. Italy has already taken this step, importing workers from Peru, as has Japan, which has turned to the Philippines.[38] We need to make sure that post-9/11 paranoia doesn't lead to cutting off our own lifeline.

Paradoxically, the conflation of sub-acute nursing home care (short-term rehabilitation) and chronic nursing home care (long-term residence) may prove to be the crucial stimulus for getting nursing homes on the public's radar screen. Almost every older person requires hospitalization sooner or later, usually multiple times during their Medicare years. Increasingly, hospital stays are truncated to such a degree that elderly patients cannot return home directly but need to stop over in a skilled nursing facility to get back on their feet. As a result, a growing number of patients and their families will have exposure to the world of nursing homes earlier than they would have in a previous era. Although many of these interim stays are brief, and the indignities of nursing home care are far more tolerable if they only last a few weeks and the patient can look forward to returning home, nevertheless the infantilization and dehumanization experienced in nursing homes are likely to leave an indelible mark.

We can hope that greater awareness of the problems of nursing home care and a recognition that it doesn't have to be this way will inspire advocacy. A robust consumer movement would add considerably to the efforts of the National Citizens' Nursing Home Reform Coalition, which at this point is focusing more on labor issues in nursing homes—staffing ratios, staff training, and staff wages—than on the quality of life of their residents. Advocacy in the form of a strengthened consumer movement will go a long way toward creating the kinds of nursing homes that the baby boomers will be willing to live in. Consumers will need to join forces with professional medical organizations to exert pressure on CMS to redesign the regulatory underpinnings of nursing homes.

Even more fundamentally, however, we need to put long-term care on the national agenda. Right now Medicare is the only program of consequence to the elderly that is in the public eye. The only widely acknowledged omission from the Medicare program has been coverage for prescription drugs, which the Medicare Modernization Act of 2003 will ostensibly remedy. In fact, as I discussed in Chapter 4, Medicare needs a much more extensive overhaul, not just the addition of a modest medication benefit. But Medicare reform, even comprehensive reform, is only part of what needs to change for every American to be assured of good care in old age. Long-term care, which encompasses nursing home care, assisted living, and home care programs, must become a topic that is debated by politicians along with homeland security and tax cuts. Politicians have deliberately stayed away from long-term care because talking about it will force them to come around to thinking about paying for it. In their view, it's bad enough that over 35 percent of the Medicaid budget goes for long-term care.[39] It's bad enough that home care has undergone explosive growth (though checked slightly by the Balanced Budget Act), with Medicaid alone spending $11.5 billion on home and community-based long-term care. Thinking in a comprehensive way about long-term care, about how to integrate the various components into a coordinated whole, is something that nobody running for elective office has dared to do. But as legislators increasingly discover that their very own parents are poorly served by the current mishmash of services that together constitute long-term care, maybe they will see the light. Perhaps what it will take is for a few brave presidential candidates to reveal their personal stories of struggling to ensure that their own family members have a dignified old age. Only then will we confront the need for fundamental change in nursing homes—their underlying philosophy, how we regulate them, their manpower needs, and a financing system that will pay for it all.

SIX

Assisted Living: Boon or Boondoggle?

W HEN THE baby boomers are asked about nursing home care, we are very consistent: we don't want any part of it. The pundits claim that nearly half of us will spend time in a nursing home before we die,[1] but we think they are mistaken. We believe we will be able to avoid nursing homes altogether—and the reason is that we will take advantage of assisted living instead.

Assisted living is more a philosophy than a well-defined entity. According to the Assisted Living Federation of America, it is "a special combination of housing, supportive services, personalized assistance, and healthcare designed to respond to the individual needs of those who require help with activities of daily living."[2] It is a label for various kinds of residences—including older homes that look like a rooming house, with private rooms and communal living and dining areas, as well as newer apartment complexes that feature studios and one-bedroom units. All told, there are 36,400 residences in the United States that call themselves assisted living, housing just over one million people. The typical resident is an 83-year-old widow, more likely white than black, and more likely paying privately. While the building she lives in could have as few as three occupants and as many as 200, the average size is 43 units. Residents of assisted living, on average, stay in the facility for close to three years, with a third moving on to a nursing home, 28 percent dying, 12 percent moving in with family members, and 14 percent switching to a different assisted living facility.[3]

According to CNN, assisted living is "the hottest new housing option for senior citizens." Older people and their anxious offspring can rest assured that in some of the new upscale retirement homes, they will find "a sense of peace, companionship, comfort, security, and belonging."[4] In 1999, *Fortune* Magazine designated assisted living as one of three potential growth industries.[5] For the first time, in the 1990s, companies that build assisted living went public: "Wall Street investors, eyeing the impending retirement of millions of baby boomers . . . fell all over themselves trying to catch a piece of the boom."[6] As a result, the number of assisted living facilities increased a stunning 49 percent between 1991 and 1999, and then another 48 percent between 1998 and 2003.[7] Terrified of nursing homes and having difficulty making it in their own homes, more and more older people are latching onto assisted living as offering the ideal mix of a residential environment, home care services, and a philosophy of consumer choice. But is it the perfect blend, or is it, as some have suggested, synonymous with "fraud, false promises, and potential neglect?"[8]

Wʜᴇɴ ᴍʏ mother-in-law was dying, she mumbled to me that her husband, Saul, would need to enter a nursing home after she was gone. She was revealing a secret she had kept for over a year: Saul had dementia. Once she was no longer around to run his life for him, to bolster his failing memory with her fully functioning mind and to compensate for his growing disorganization, the secret would become public knowledge. Following her death, Saul managed without her for a while, relying more and more extensively on a gentle and devoted woman who served as a combination housekeeper, personal attendant, and companion. My husband made the trip from Boston to Philadelphia each month to pay bills, set up appointments, and check up on his father.

The way we learned what was really going on with Saul during this transitional period was through the diary he kept, which he eagerly showed my husband. Always a methodical and conscientious person and a pharmacist by profession, he had gotten into the habit of keeping a medication record. He wrote down what pills he took and when, and then began embellishing the diary with notations about medical symptoms: he reported on his bowels and his sinuses, their quirks and their triumphs. Next he began documenting what he ate for each meal, along with all sorts of curious entries penned in an increasingly lopsided script. When the notes revealed that Saul was subsisting primarily on ice cream and cookies, which he apparently consumed at midnight or five A.ᴍ., and that he either took his blood pressure medicine twice as often as prescribed or not at all, the time had clearly come to move him to a more supervised setting.

Contrary to my mother-in-law's expectations, Saul did not enter a nursing home. Instead, we persuaded him to move into assisted living. Saul would have a one-bedroom apartment in a sparkling, newly renovated building. He would have three balanced meals a day at the conventional times in an elegant dining room, where attentive young waitresses would serve him. A housekeeper would clean his apartment weekly, and he would be able to go to movies and musical recitals on the premises. In short, he would have all the help he needed without sacrificing privacy or dignity. My husband and I found an assisted living residence a few miles from our home so that our visits could be far more frequent—and less onerous—than the monthly treks to Philadelphia. We were ecstatic, and Saul was only slightly less so.

Six months later, my husband and I were no longer ecstatic, although Saul had adjusted remarkably well and had even found a lady friend. Saul was still missing meals—he forgot to go to the dining room unless his friend reminded him. He did not care for the orderly who tried to give him a shower each day, and his personal hygiene suffered as a result. He was getting more confused: he sometimes mistook the communal television room for his own apartment and, oblivious to all the proper ladies dozing in their seats, began undressing for bed. We learned of these issues when the assisted living director notified us that unless these problems were rectified, Saul would need to find a new home.

Our experience with the world of assisted living was profoundly disappointing. The facility was unequipped to provide the ongoing monitoring and supervision necessary for individuals with cognitive impairment. It paid lip service to the idea of allowing its residents to "age in place"—to provide more assistance as they developed more problems—but when the residents became frail, it was ready to boot them out. When we tried to find a solution, we uncovered further flaws in what had seemed like the perfect arrangement. The facility agreed, for an additional fee, to provide reminders before each meal. But the staff members doing the reminding had no intuitive sense about how to interact with cognitively impaired people and no compensatory training. The young woman assigned to tell Saul that it would soon be lunchtime banged on his apartment door forty-five minutes before lunch was served, which was thirty minutes too early. She barked brusquely that he should get ready for lunch and left. Within fifteen minutes, he had managed to forget the unpleasant encounter—and that it was lunchtime.

We tried to arrange for an aide to give Saul his pills, since his medication consumption was at best erratic and at worst dangerous, as it had been when he lived alone at home. Because assisted living is not a "medical" facility, we were told, staff members were not allowed to administer the medicine. An aide could tell Saul to take his pills, but she could not actually remove the pill from a bottle and hand it to him. When the aide told him it was pill time—the same aide who reminded him it was mealtime—he routinely responded that he would take his pills "later." The insistence that "Golden Acres"[9] was not a medical facility also made it difficult to evaluate Saul's incontinence and memory. The assisted living facility boasted that it had a registered nurse on site three days a week. However, she was instructed not to speak to a resident's physician to provide first-hand information about his symptoms. Instead, her role was strictly to serve as a middleman: she called us to say there was a problem, which she described in vague, non-clinical terms since we were family members, and suggested that we contact Saul's physician.

Our experience with assisted living also brought home to us just how expensive this "all-inclusive" option could be. The $3,000 per month rent covered room and meals plus half an hour of personal care (the morning shower) each day. Everything else was à la carte: the mealtime reminders, ineffective as they were, generated an additional charge. Each reminder was billed as taking half an hour, most of which was consumed by "travel time" (the ride on the elevator to and from the apartment) and by "documentation" (writing down that the aide took the elevator, went to the apartment, and told Saul to go to lunch). The recording typically took up more time than the actual reminding. Laundry service was not part of the "comprehensive package," though it, too, was available at a price. Saul's hygiene issues necessitated supplementary housecleaning services, in particular bathroom cleaning and linen changing, three times a week, not the customary once weekly—also available for a fee. Each month a professional billing company sent us an itemized accounting of the many "services" Saul received—until we decided that the vaunted "privacy" was a euphemism for "neglect" and transferred him yet again, this time to a nursing home.

CONTRARY to the prevailing wisdom, assisted living is not a new concept. The idea of a home that simultaneously affords privacy and offers a modest amount of assistance has been around for more than a century. In fact, rest homes, which were essentially rooming houses for the elderly, were the predecessors of contemporary nursing homes. Their evolution from largely unregulated mom-and-pop institutions to bureaucratic, rigid nursing homes is as instructive as it is disturbing. Rest homes, also called old age homes, were first created in the latter part of the nineteenth century as a reaction against the almshouse, previously the only source of institutional care for poor elderly people unable to care for themselves. Old age homes, by contrast, were designed to provide care to the "worthy poor," treating them with the respect and dignity that were invariably lacking in almshouses.

Old age homes at the end of the nineteenth century tended to be small and intimate. In the greater Boston area, the median occupancy was 29, with all but two facilities housing fewer than 60 residents.[10] They were culturally homogeneous, typically catering to a particular ethnic or religious group: for example, there were the Swedish Home and the German Home (whose institutional descendants survive today as long-term-care facilities). The Burnap Free Home for Aged Women was established in 1901 for elderly Protestant women; the German Ladies Aid Society was built in 1893 for "indigent Germans"; and the Baptist Home started out in 1892 in Cambridge, Massachusetts, as an abode for "deserving" but ailing Baptists.[11]

Like today's assisted living facilities, the nineteenth-century old age homes were not medically oriented. They expected their residents to be reasonably healthy. Admission was contingent on certification by a physician that the individual was able to care for herself and for her room. Physicians and nurses attended to the needs of the residents, but the care was supervised by—and to a large extent provided by—a matron, who in turn reported to the board of the home. As the minutes of the board of the Roxbury Home for Aged Women record, "our dear old ladies must receive every attention necessary to their comfort," and if the matron did not provide it, she would be fired. The focus was on quality of life; the homes recognized that familiar food, a common language, and celebration of shared holidays were essential. In general, these homes believed in what is now called "aging in place": the average length of stay at one typical facility was 13.3 years.[12]

Old age homes developed largely in response to the inadequacies of the poorhouses that increasingly served as a repository for the elderly.[13] In addition to being dirty, corrupt, and often brutal, almshouses failed to attend to the emotional and social needs of their inmates. Public welfare reformers advocated, with some degree of success, for improved conditions in almshouses, but it was private sectarian groups, not wanting to wait for reforms to be instituted, who developed non-profit homes to provide a homier, less institutional environment for needy elders.

These informally organized establishments were headed for trouble, however, precisely because they conceived of themselves as homes, not hospitals. Fire destroyed a number of facilities, killing residents who were not completely mobile. The homes occasionally had problems with cleanliness and safety, and the food was sometimes neither tasty nor nutritious. The 1950s ushered in an era of regulation of rest homes, with state licensing requirements mandating changes in sanitation, ventilation, and staffing. As rest homes struggled to remain financially viable in an age of growing regulation, they also faced stiff competition from the new nursing home industry. Stimulated by the federal Hill-Burton Act of 1954, which granted public money for building nursing homes, new large facilities modeled on hospitals sprang up. The final blow to the rest home movement was the passage of Medicaid in 1965, which paid for the care of poor people in licensed nursing facilities. A few rest homes survived, renamed board and care facilities, appealing as they always had to older people who were alone in the world, too independent to require a nursing home, but for whom staying in a house or apartment was a lonely, burdensome prospect. They typically offered a private room, often though not always a private bath, weekly housekeeping, and communal meals. It is these rest homes that are the common ancestor of both the assisted living facility and the nursing home of today.

Like their nineteenth-century predecessors, assisted living facilities today work best for those who need a little help getting up in the morning, primarily with washing and dressing, and then again in the evening, essentially reversing the earlier routine. In between these two allotments of care, the individual must be able to function on her own. Ideally, she should be able to get herself to the dining room on schedule three times a day for meals. She should be able to keep a copy of the facility's calendar of events so she can choose the activities she wants to attend. Moreover, when she is alone in her apartment, reveling in the privacy that assisted living so proudly provides, she must be able to manage. A selling point of assisted living is the kitchen facilities in each apartment, so that residents will be able to make a cup of tea whenever they choose, but if a resident leaves the kettle on the stove long after all the water has boiled away, then she cannot cope with an unmonitored environment. If she is incontinent—and an estimated 21 percent of assisted living residents were incontinent in a study done in 1999, with the proportion growing yearly—she has to be capable of changing her adult diapers and washing out her underwear, and must at least be free of bowel incontinence.

Assisted living begins to break down when cognitive impairment is severe enough that a person needs frequent reminders so as not to miss meals. It disintegrates further when the resident has to be told every few hours to go to the bathroom in order to decrease the risk of incontinence. The problem with Alzheimer's disease and other dementias is that they demand almost constant vigilance. It would be florid neglect to leave a two-year-old unattended for hours at a time, and it is just as absurd to think that a person with all but the mildest dementia can be left alone in his apartment. Dementia by definition entails poor judgment and difficulty in problem-solving. Only another person with a fully intact mind can compensate for such deficits.[14]

Despite these concerns, assisted living facilities not only are home to a large number of people with dementia, but in many cases they advertise that they are uniquely designed for demented residents. Have such specialized facilities overcome the inadequacies of conventional, all-purpose assisted living? Or are the claims about offering a secure home for the memory-impaired merely a marketing ploy? A *Time* magazine article tells the horror story of an elderly woman, Dorothy, who moved to an assisted living facility in Minnesota, owned and operated by the for-profit giant,

Alterra. The woman's son, Peter, was attracted to Alterra Clare Bridge, a residence for the memory-impaired, from the moment he saw the facility; from the outside, he said, it "looked more like a resort than a hospital." He found the concept of assisted living tremendously appealing: it was "a new way to live—and die—with dignity and freedom." He liked the town square he encountered when he entered the building, which boasted a beauty salon, an ice cream parlor, and a large living room with a fireplace. What he learned, however, was that the only "enrichment" in which his mother participated, when left to her own devices (which was all the time), was watching television. Unable to cut her toenails, unaware that they needed cutting, and unable to articulate that she needed help, Dorothy went eight months without a podiatrist, until her nails "grew so long that they circled over the tops of her toes."[15]

Peter's experience is not an isolated case. A careful study of assisted living and residential care across four states found that many facilities claimed they had a dementia-specific program, but by all the measures the investigators used, they were unable to distinguish between the dementia care programs and the regular programs.[16] Conceivably, because all assisted living facilities have residents with dementia, usually in excess of 35 percent of their clientele, they all have developed excellent ways of caring for people with cognitive impairment. More likely, none of them has. The special services and tailored programs ostensibly available at dementia care facilities are no more successful than the standard fare in addressing the need for continuous supervision.

A few facilities reportedly have come up with ways to simultaneously provide a homey environment for people with dementia and to discreetly keep an eye on them. Evergreen in Oshkosh, Wisconsin, for instance, has developed a model of assisted living for people with dementia that is really a group home. In fact, it is closer to a good nursing home—one that truly respects individuals and affords them privacy and dignity—than to assisted living. The building consists of private rooms that are left open for purposes of surveillance and cozy communal spaces that are continually monitored. As long as the residents do not have major physical disabilities, they can be accommodated in the complex. European institutions have likewise developed "therapeutic environments" that both support and challenge residents. Individuals with dementia remain in these facilities indefinitely, only entering a nursing home if they become severely impaired or develop behavioral problems.[17]

For assisted living to be a viable option for people with dementia, it will need to be structured very differently from the usual "special care" facility. Perhaps what we need is not assisted living at all, but instead radically redesigned nursing homes in which privacy and autonomy are respected. Only the latter are able to provide the round-the-clock assistance, reminders, and monitoring which people with dementia need. The challenge is to develop institutions that do all this in a manner that acknowledges, respects, and responds to each individual person.

Assisted living was perfect for Ellen Taft. She had had polio as a child, and after retiring from teaching music, she developed post-polio syndrome. Her legs, which had always been slightly weak, were now less reliable than ever. One was shorter and more deformed than the other. She had limped since childhood, but now Ellen wore a heavy metal brace on the short leg and used a walker to maintain her balance. Widowed at age 60, she had continued to live in the three-story Victorian house where she had brought up her three children. Upkeep of the house, with its built-in dust-gathering bookcases, ornate wooden inlay, and spiral staircase, was too much for Ellen. With her children long gone, dispersed across the country, she had no need for four bedrooms. She hadn't held a dinner party in years and only ate in the dining room when her children brought Thanksgiving dinner to her. Moreover, Ellen was lonely. Most of her friends had died or moved to Florida. She mused that the only reason for staying in the house was her 1927 Mason & Hamlin grand piano.

Ellen decided that it was time to move after she fell in the kitchen while reaching for a can of soup. The soup was tantalizingly close, on a shelf just above eye level. She lost her balance reaching for it and ended up on the floor, unable to stand or to get to the telephone. Her daughter discovered her four hours later when she arrived to take her out to dinner. Instead of spending the evening in a restaurant, they spent it in the local hospital emergency room. Miraculously, Ellen had not broken her hip or any other bones. She was sent home with little more than instructions to be careful, to take Tylenol for her bruises, and to return to the hospital if she failed to improve in some unspecified period of time. Her daughter, Geraldine, stayed with her overnight and was preparing to discuss getting a Life Line monitor and a housekeeper, but Ellen preempted her.

She declared in her usual authoritative way that she planned to move. The house was old and falling apart, and she would prefer to live someplace brighter and more modern. Geraldine was stunned. She had expected a fight; she had been convinced that her mother would never leave her home of sixty years and that the best she could hope for was that she would accept a little help.

Ellen surprised her daughter again a month later by announcing that not only did she plan to move, but she had already found a suitable new home and would be moving in shortly. Geraldine had anticipated some degree of backsliding from the original decision and a certain amount of procrastinating. She had not realized her mother would apply her single-mindedness and determination to the problem of choosing an assisted living facility, just as she had to selecting private schools for her children or making a career as a pianist. Ellen set a date for the move. Given that she was going from ten rooms to three, she expected her children to help her pack what little she could take with her and keep what they wanted for themselves. The rest they would have to dispose of. She would, of course, supervise the packing and the distribution. The house would go to her oldest son, Max, who was trying, not very successfully, to earn a living as a tennis pro, and who could use either a place to live or the not inconsequential proceeds from selling the house. He also had the time to attend to fixing the house so that it could be put on the market and to deal with lawyers, realtors, and banks.

Two months after the fall, Ellen Taft moved into a boxy one-bedroom apartment in Central Towers, a complex located only a mile from her previous home. She liked the idea that she would be able to stay in contact with the few friends who still lived in the area and that she wouldn't feel she was going to unknown territory. Her unit in the five-story building overlooked the busy street below. She had a bedroom that was barely large enough for a bed and a night table, a living room that looked cramped as soon as her plump velour sofa and matching armchair arrived, along with her cherry dining room table, a wedding gift from her parents. The apartment also featured a kitchenette with all the usual appliances in diminutive versions. The only room that had clearly been designed with its future clientele in mind was the bathroom, which was wheelchair-accessible, with grab bars next to the toilet and a walk-in shower with a low ledge at the entrance.

Ellen didn't plan to spend much time in her apartment, so its simple utilitarian construction didn't faze her. Once her son Max mounted several of her favorite prints on the walls and she lined up photos of her children on the windowsills, it looked homey enough. Ellen lingered in the dining room during meals, regaling anyone who would listen with tales of her exploits and with political commentary.

She was one of the few residents who made use of the library's small and eclectic collection of books. Ellen surmised that the books had been given by the children of tenants at the time of their death, though conceivably some of them were donated when new residents moved in and found they didn't have sufficient space in their own apartments. She also made liberal use of the Towers' grand piano, located conspicuously in the first-floor sitting room. It wasn't nearly as nice as hers and it needed to be tuned—but Ellen complained loudly enough that a piano tuner showed up within a few days of her arrival.

Ellen thrived at the Towers. Relieved of the tedium of shopping, cooking, and cleaning, which she had found all-consuming and exhausting, she went to all the movies the facility offered: a few old classics and a great many recently released videos. She listened to every outside speaker. She used the Towers as her base of operation, arranging for trips to museums, to concerts downtown, and to medical appointments, with the van driver from "The Ride" picking her up and returning her home.

At age 80, Ellen was a little younger than the average resident of assisted living, who is typically 83. Like her peers, she needed help in a few basic activities such as bathing and dressing, but was more independent than her counterparts in nursing homes. Like other assisted living residents, she was better educated than most people in her age cohort. Like all the other residents of the Towers and most assisted living residents nationwide, she was far more affluent than the majority of octogenarians. And like the ideal assisted living resident, she was not so sick as to need help the facility was not designed to provide, and because her mind was perfectly clear, she could plan and organize her days. A half-hour of personal care in the morning and in the evening, three meals a day, and housekeeping services were just what she needed. On-site activities, principally in the form of speakers and movies, were an added bonus, particularly during the long Boston winters when it was hard for her to get out.

Ellen may have flourished at the Towers, but within a month she was devoting most of her mealtime conversation to trenchant critiques of the staff, the management, and the physical plant. For the most part, she was as insightful as she was devastating in her assessments. First of all, she observed, the Towers did not have enough staff. Aides were assigned to help the majority of the residents get dressed and ready for breakfast. They started at 6:30 A.M., but if they spent half an hour with each resident they would not be finished until ten, and breakfast was over at nine. In a similar vein, the Towers sent aides to remind selected residents to go to lunch. In order to get to everyone with the available staff, they had to begin the reminding at 10:30, which gave the residents ample time to forget before noon, when lunch actually started. This wasn't as bad as the situation at some other assisted living facilities, however. One extremely unfortunate incident uncovered by investigative reporters involved an elderly woman who wandered outside in the midst of a heat wave. All but one of the facility's staff members were in a meeting. Nobody noticed the resident leave, and no one missed her—she was found about an hour later, unconscious, with a body temperature of 108 degrees. She was transported to a local hospital, where she was determined to be dead on arrival.[18]

Not only did the Towers not have enough employees, Ellen insisted, but the ones they had were inadequately trained. She had observed a man who lived down the hall from her choke on his food at dinnertime. Not one of the wait staff had a clue as to what to do. If the son of another resident hadn't happened to be visiting and performed the Heimlich maneuver, the poor man would probably have choked to death.[19] Sometimes Ellen took matters into her own hands. A woman who often ate at the same table with Ellen began missing meals. When she did make it to the dining room, she was confused and had trouble finding words. Ellen mentioned to the Towers director that her tablemate didn't seem to be herself, but the director assured her that "sometimes our residents get like that."[20] A day later, her speech was slurred and she had difficulty walking. Ellen boldly rifled through her handbag to find her wallet, extracted the name and telephone number of the woman's daughter, and promptly called her. Skeptical but anxious, the daughter showed up within an hour. She took one look at her mother, who had been completely coherent and impeccably coiffed the previous weekend and who was now inarticulate and disheveled, and called 911. At the hospital, the emergency room physician discovered that the woman's sodium level was dangerously elevated. After a couple of days of intravenous treatment, she was back to normal. Ellen worried about her when she didn't come back to the Towers, but heard through the grapevine that she had moved in with her daughter until they could find a new place for her to live.

When Ellen Taft took her daughter Miranda on a tour of the common areas at the Towers, she delivered a non-stop commentary on every person and every room they encountered. She was, as Miranda would say later, the perfect anti–tour guide. "They have these huge potted plants to make the place look nice," Ellen observed. "But they're blocking the entrance to the living room, so it's hard to get in if you're using a wheelchair." They passed one of the waitresses on her way to the dining room. "She's really fresh. Always has a smart-aleck answer for everything." And then, on noticing one of the chefs heading into the kitchen: "The food here is so salty, it's a wonder we don't all go into heart failure. One of the women I sit with is supposed to have a low-salt diet, another one's on a diabetic diet, and a third one is supposed to watch her cholesterol. But we all get the same thing at each meal. And I can guarantee you that the beef noodle soup followed by macaroni and cheese is not a low-sodium, low-cholesterol, low-carbohydrate lunch."

The most dangerous feature of the Towers, Ellen explained to her daughter, was that they accepted tenants who were too sick for them to take proper care of. "It's not just that I don't like it when the woman behind me continually asks what's going on at every movie," she said, although clearly she found the chatter intensely annoying. "And it's more than just that man who forgets where he is every evening and starts taking his clothes off in the community room. The people who've lost their marbles have to be watched all the time, and they aren't. One of these days someone's going to make himself a cup of tea and set the whole place on fire." Not only did many of the tenants suffer from dementia, but they had serious physical problems as well. One man was on blood-thinning medication and had to receive messages from his doctor's office about what dose to take, depending on the results of his blood tests. He couldn't hear very well, and he didn't have an answering machine in his apartment. The Towers felt it couldn't serve as the middleman between the patient and his doctor, so half the time the messages never reached him. Finally, the doctor decided he was better off without the medicine, risking a stroke rather than chancing a hemorrhage from too much medication.[21]

Ellen finished the tour by showing her daughter a man in a wheelchair, gazing vacantly across the room. "He sits all day. He never moves. He has a bag to catch his urine. A couple of times a day, someone comes and empties the bag. He doesn't even get out of his chair at mealtimes. That little cushion he sits on isn't going to protect his skin from ulcerating." And then she said forcefully, "If I ever get that bad, promise you'll get me out of here."

ASSISTED living is not likely to be a panacea for individuals with dementia, and it won't be much help for most people unless its financing is drastically altered. The median income for people over age 65 in 2003 was $20,363 for men and $11,845 for women, and the average annual cost of assisted living was $30,288, which does not include Medicare premiums or personal items.[22] But assisted living will not be of interest to anybody if the regulatory issues are not properly addressed. Right now, in most states, assisted living is minimally regulated, with care ranging from unsatisfactory to downright abusive and negligent. But the rules to ensure quality have the potential of either driving corporations out of business or recreating all the rigid, dehumanizing, institutional features that plague nursing homes. For assisted living to become the highly desirable option that many older people wish it were, state regulators will need to exhibit an uncommon degree of imagination and responsiveness to advocacy groups.

The media are full of stories of what happens when assisted living goes unregulated. In New York State, with virtually no rules governing who can run an assisted living facility, what training staff members must have, and what services must be offered, the Health Department regularly gets complaints about residents who wander outside at night, who are left unattended, and who develop pressure ulcers.[23] The largest assisted living chain, Alterra, owner of the facility where Dorothy lived, was investigated in at least five states. Its accusers claimed that the staff members at Alterra's facilities were untrained, that it failed to ensure that elderly residents got the pills that had been prescribed for them, and that what little it did to keep its residents safe was grossly inadequate.

In California, regulators sought to revoke the license of nine facilities run by another chain, Regent Assisted Living. The stimulus was the death of a 79-year-old woman who bled to death in her rocking chair, allegedly after several calls for help went unanswered. A federal government report on assisted living noted that even when regulations did exist, facilities violated them with impunity. Fully 27 percent of the facilities surveyed had been cited for more than five quality-of-care violations over a two-year period.[24] And a prominent researcher in the long-term care field commented that "most states require more training for manicurists and dog groomers than for assisted living caregivers."[25]

The industry responded to charges of negligence by claiming it had a private understanding with regulators that whatever rules existed would be relaxed to "accommodate an aging in place philosophy."[26] The industry also claims that the horror stories that make the newspapers are rare exceptions, not routine occurrences. But in response to escalating insurance costs and pressure to increase the size of the staff, several assisted living chains have declared bankruptcy, and others have simply sold off the assisted living piece of their business. In 2002, for instance, Marriott, which had entered the assisted living market with considerable fanfare, promising to bring its "hospitality" orientation to the dreary world of long-term care, pulled out. The Milwaukee-based Alterra Corporation spent a billion dollars on restructuring in a desperate attempt to stave off bankruptcy. Its revenues fell 22 percent between 2001 and 2002—and in the end, the company filed for Chapter 11.[27] Financial hard times in that period were not conducive to bolstering staff training and numbers or to adding more recreational activities and personal care services.

The idea that regulations would ensure quality care in assisted living surfaced after a study by the General Accounting Office (GAO) in 1999 turned up evidence of major deficiencies in assisted living. The GAO found so many differences between assisted living facilities that comparing quality proved impossible. It also noted inadequate staffing levels, reports of neglect and abuse, and extensive complaints by residents. In response, assisted living facilities promised to go through an accreditation process. Two years later, on reviewing progress in the industry, the U.S. Senate Special Committee on Aging found that there had been none. As a result, the committee's chairman, John Breaux, asked the Consumer Consortium on Assisted Living, a national, non-profit organization dedicated to advocating for assisted living consumers, to put together a group to develop recommendations for improving quality. The ensuing work group consisted of 48 organizations, including consumers, regulators, health care providers, and assisted living operators. It was an excellent idea, but the group's report, released in the spring of 2003, was a disappointment.[28] The authors of the study could not even agree on a definition of assisted living. The majority defined assisted living by its philosophy, not by what it delivers. The report emphasized "the right to make choices and to receive services in a way that will promote the resident's dignity, autonomy, independence, and quality of life." Dissenters responded bluntly that "this feel-good language does nothing to inform a consumer" about just what services he can rely on.

In a similar vein, the work group's report listed eight "core principles" that should "guide" any assisted living facility. These included assertions that the facility should "provide resident-centered services" that focus on the specific needs of each individual and that it should "minimize the need to move." The dissenters argued that these principles are "at best . . . aspiration statements." They described them as marketing principles that bear no relationship to the concrete recommendations in the report: "We believe the core principles are misleading" and "should not have been included in the report."

Several of the original participants in the Consortium on Assisted Living were so dissatisfied that they wrote their own report.[29] These groups included the National Citizens' Coalition for Nursing Home Reform, a non-profit organization that began as an offshoot of the Gray Panthers and has over 200 organizational members and 1,000 individual members, and the National Senior Citizens' Law Center, a legal advocacy group that focuses primarily on poor, disabled elders. This second report stated the case for regulations clearly and succinctly. First, the groups observed that it is no longer true that assisted living is housing for fundamentally healthy older people; the population served by assisted living is becoming almost indistinguishable from the nursing home population. They summarized the problems reported in assisted living, such as undiagnosed and untreated medical problems, malnutrition, and wandering, and concluded that they stem from inadequate training of staff and insufficient monitoring and supervision of residents. To assure good quality of care, they proposed defining two or more levels of care and stating explicitly what services are provided at each level of care. Standard staffing ratios and training requirements should be established for each level, and uniform public health and safety standards (for example, fire codes) should be mandated for all assisted living facilities. Finally, the report emphasized the need for federal oversight of state standards, at least for all facilities accepting Medicaid. In short, the report called for exactly the same sort of federal control over the assisted living industry as is currently exerted over the nursing home industry.

The fear, as others are quick to point out, is that such rules will regiment and bureaucratize the lives of residents, just as regulations did in nursing homes. Realistically, the solution to the problem of quality control in assisted living facilities will almost undoubtedly include specific rules, since altruism and beneficence have historically been insufficient to guarantee quality. Moreover, the largely for-profit, corporate world of assisted living is more likely to be characterized by avarice and greed than by beneficence. But is there any reason why the rules cannot be crafted so as to support rather than undermine the philosophy of assisted living? Surely regulations do not make it impossible to respect an older person's dignity, to afford him privacy, and to tailor his "care plan" to his particular needs and interests.

Consider the recommendation that assisted living facilities

adopt standard staffing ratios. Presumably, the numbers of staff per resident would vary depending on the level of impairment of the population served. There is no inherent reason why quantifying how many people should be on site will have a deleterious effect on the spirit of a facility. What *would* be problematic is to require that the people who provide care be of particular types—nurses, nurse's aides, home health attendants. Utilizing traditional categories works against creating holistic helpers. Far more conducive to establishing a homelike atmosphere than division of labor would be the widespread use of multi-purpose personnel or "universal workers." In a family, after all, the daughter may be the one who changes bandages and the son the one who deals with the accountants and the lawyers, but if grandma needs a prescription picked up from the pharmacy, whoever is available will get it for her. Narrowly defined job descriptions in assisted living can have a stultifying effect if workers regularly refuse to be helpful on the grounds that "it's not my job." But while assisted living facilities should feel free to determine for themselves what kinds of frontline caregivers they need, and should be encouraged to cross-train workers so they can perform many different kinds of service, there is no reason they cannot be obligated by law to have an established minimum staffing ratio.

The suggestion that all assisted living facilities provide on-the-job training for employees seems likewise unobjectionable. Learning how to deal with problems such as incontinence and dementia can only improve the quality of care in assisted living facilities. In fact, wait staff and receptionists are just as desperately in need of this kind of education as are nurse's aides. When my father-in-law was in assisted living, he was deeply offended by the rudeness of many of the waitresses—and warmly enthusiastic when he encountered a kind and friendly one. More often than not, the wait staff took his plate away before he was finished eating. They forgot to bring him the beverage he requested and then accused him of having imagined he had asked for it. They routinely spoke too softly to residents with impaired hearing. Naturally, the content of training sessions has to be carefully chosen. If the focus is exclusively on health and safety, if staff members are not taught that residents sometimes value autonomy more than health, then training will undermine the assisted living philosophy. But a requirement that all staff members undergo a few hours of training before they start and then once a year thereafter is hardly objectionable or excessively burdensome.

A final recommendation of the dissenting work group is that facilities offer at least two discrete levels of care. Each level necessitates particular services: the lower level of care, for instance, might include transportation to medical appointments in a facility van and a registered nurse on site 12 hours a week. The higher level of care might require a nurse on site 24 hours a week, administration of medication in residents' apartments, and a nutritionist to provide special diets for residents with certain medical needs (low-salt diets for people with heart failure, a diet without concentrated sweets for individuals with diabetes, low-cholesterol diets for people with coronary artery disease, and so on). The notion that assisted living should not provide on-site medical care because that would "medicalize" the facility is foolish. If the facility chose to administer medications to its residents by having them all line up before breakfast to get their medicine, it would be guilty of excessive medicalization, or more precisely of creating an institutional environment. It would certainly be engaging in medicalization if it chose to solve the problem of administering medication by hiring a nurse in a starched white uniform to push a medication cart around the dining room in order to deliver pills, as in a hospital. Most people who take medications on a regular basis do so in the privacy of their homes, typically at the kitchen table with a glass of water. The assisted living facility ought to enable them to do exactly that, which would mean training staff to go to the apartment at specified times, engage the resident in conversation, perhaps have a cup of tea, and in the course of the visit, give the medication. Requiring that facilities offer the kinds of services needed by residents who have a significant burden of disease and disability would only lead to regimentation if the assisted living facility implemented the regulation inappropriately. The facilities should have no discretion about what services are provided, but a great deal of choice about how they are delivered.

Just as the regulations proposed by the dissenting work group members can be implemented without destroying the mission of assisted living, so too can the linchpin of the majority report, the negotiated risk contract, be instituted without devastating consequences. In fact, the negotiated risk contract, if properly drawn up and adhered to, could very well protect both operators and residents of assisted living. The motivation for such contracts is the tension between safety and autonomy in the lives of older people: regulated facilities are at risk of being penalized for failing to monitor residents adequately—regardless of whether the resident was willing to be monitored. The concept of negotiated risk essentially gets the facility off the hook in the event that there are adverse consequences of a resident's personal decision making. If a diabetic resident chooses to eat sweets and develops uncontrolled diabetes, the facility should not be penalized for serving cake at a birthday celebration; if a resident decides to use a cane because he refuses to be seen in public with a walker, and then falls and breaks his wrist, the assisted living residence should not be held accountable for excessive falls. The negotiated risk contract specifies what the facility will offer—diabetic diets, physical therapy consultation—and what aspects of his life the resident takes responsibility for. By addressing the liability issue, facilities feel more comfortable respecting the autonomy of residents. But skeptics argue that negotiated risk contracts, far from allowing a facility to honor a resident's preferences, are actually a means of allowing an assisted living facility to "admit or retain a resident whose needs the facility cannot meet, and . . . [have] the resident release the facility from any liability arising from the facility's inadequate care."[30]

I use something very similar to negotiated risk all the time in clinical practice. In the office, if I propose a treatment that is less aggressive than maximal medical care—such as treating someone's angina with medications rather than with angioplasty—I discuss the pros and cons of the various alternatives. In particular, I make very clear that the alternative therapy is apt to be less effective than its more aggressive counterpart, but that it comes with a different array of side effects. If it's important enough to the patient to stay out of the hospital and to avoid surgery, then she may be willing to accept a lower probability of success in exchange for treatment that avoids precisely what she most fears. That constitutes negotiating risk—with the implicit understanding that the patient is not going to sue later on for my failing to provide the "best" treatment. The same sort of negotiation works in assisted living (and in both cases, the substance of the discussion must be written down). For example, a resident might benefit from help with bathing, but she finds the prospect of "being showered" by an aide an affront to her dignity. The facility can try to find a way to maximize her safety *and* respect her dignity, perhaps by suggesting baths rather than showers or by finding a different aide with whom she feels more comfortable. If the resident finds these alternatives unsatisfactory, insists on bathing independently, and falls in the bathroom, the facility should not be considered negligent.

Of course, negotiated risk contracts cannot be an excuse for failing to provide essential services. Nor can they be flouted—in New York State, for instance, investigators found that residents were "allowed" to ignore their diabetic diets, but if they did, their families were notified (without their permission) and they were threatened with expulsion. And assisted living programs should not be directing administrators to "get" a negotiated risk contract signed whenever a resident falls, wanders off the premises, or has skin breakdown for the express purpose of trying to exonerate facilities from negligent behavior.[31] But if the contracts are meaningful—if residents understand what they are agreeing to and if the facility truly honors the agreements—they can be an important means for translating the philosophy of resident-centered care into practice.

Aʂsɪsᴛᴇᴅ living is successful principally for those elders who are cognitively intact, but only if they have money. If this is to be a reasonable option for more than a small minority of older people, financing will need to change. Right now the overwhelming majority of people in assisted living pay with their own resources. And they pay an average of $2,524 per month—in many cases, considerably more. Dorothy, the woman with the unsatisfactory experience at Clare Bridge in Eagan, Minnesota, hardly a community with the highest cost of living in the country, paid $3,450 a month, and that was in 1999. The monthly fee in 2003 for a one-bedroom unit in a city like Boston could be as high as $5,600.[32] The fee includes rent, utilities, and meals, as well as whatever personal care is provided, typically half an hour twice a day. It does not include medical expenses (such as Medicare Part B premiums or supplementary medical insurance), and it does not cover personal expenses such as clothes or the barber.

Medicaid, the insurance program for the poor, may pay for assisted living either through Supplementary Social Security Insurance (SSI) or with special waiver plans. In 2003, 41 states offered partial reimbursement to assisted living facilities for poor residents through one or the other of these approaches.[33] SSI payments can be used toward room and board; Medicaid then reimburses for the services (homemaker, home health aide) that are part of the assisted living package. The level of reimbursement is so low, however, that most assisted living facilities will not accept

Medicaid, and those that do generally restrict the percentage of units that they will fill with residents on Medicaid. The net effect was that as of 2003, only 101,000 of the nearly one million people living in assisted living were Medicaid recipients.[34]

The solution is to recognize that a neat distinction between "medical and "social" needs as people age is impossible. What older people with disabilities require, whether those disabilities arise from dementia, from heart disease, from arthritis, or from a mixture of multiple conditions, is long-term care. Or, to use the more politically correct phrase, they need long-term "supportive services."[35] Because of their health problems, these elders require a living environment that enables them to cope with their deficits. The doorways have to be wide enough to accommodate a wheelchair; the walls should have railings; the bathrooms ought to have raised toilet seats and grab bars. Wall clocks must have large, easily visible numbers; hallways have to be light enough to permit residents to find their way without tripping. Offering oxygen for people with trouble breathing but not hearing aids for people with trouble hearing nor a home health aide for someone with trouble bathing is completely arbitrary.

In order to meet the combined social and housing needs of older people, we need to add a comprehensive long-term care component to Medicare. One way to achieve this would be through a new Medicare benefit. The benefit would offer long-term care, whether at home, in an assisted living facility, or in a nursing home, to people over age 65 who need help in at least two activities of daily living. It might pay 80 percent of the cost after a $10,000 deductible, analogous to the Medicare fee schedule for physicians' services, up to a maximum of $200,000. Once the total pool was exhausted, individuals would have to pay out of pocket or use private long-term-care insurance. Medicaid would be available for those without the requisite resources. The new benefit would be financed by contributions to a trust fund, perhaps from a special payroll tax or from the Federal Estate and Gift Tax. The best estimates indicate that if we rolled out such a program today, half the benefits would be available in ten years and the entire benefit in twenty years.[36]

Ideally, we would combine Medicare and Medicaid into a single program to prevent cost-shifting between the two. But both plans—a long-term-care benefit and a merger of Medicare and Medicaid—would be expensive. These changes will require extraordinary political will—or maybe just a handful of senators and representatives with aging parents who would be ideal candidates for assisted living if only they could afford it. As a temporary measure, every state should subsidize Medicaid beneficiaries who are eligible for assisted living. They should also offer incentives to assisted living complexes to decrease their reliance on private-pay tenants. With occupancy rates down as a result of overbuilding in the late 1990s, "scholarship" residents should suddenly be quite attractive, at least compared with empty apartments.

WE HAVE seen that assisted living, at least in its current form, is not a panacea for older people who are unable to make it at home but are loath to enter a nursing home. It is improperly designed to care for people with dementia, essentially unavailable to all but the most affluent, and insufficiently regulated to provide for residents who have any significant degree of physical impairment. I have proposed various solutions—expanding Medicaid coverage for assisted living, creating a long-term-care benefit within Medicare, and developing regulations for assisted living facilities. But what would make even more sense is to recognize that the distinction between assisted living and nursing home care is at best artificial and at worst pernicious. The few assisted living facilities that work well for older people with significant physical or cognitive impairments look just like what a nursing home would look like if it were truly first-rate, if it were designed to be resident-centered. It would not necessarily resemble the gleaming apartment complexes that pass for assisted living and that are satisfactory only for the most independent older people. What we should strive for instead is three   ls of long-term care, all of which should be paid for by t   mechanisms. The lowest level of care would be very si   at much of assisted living is today: private apartm   communal dining, on-site activities, and a minimum   int of personal care. The next level of care, suitable for the largest number of people, would encompass the more dependent elders who currently live in assisted living and the less dependent of those who currently live in nursing homes. There would be private rooms and private bathrooms, but more staff members with more training, a greater degree of personal care and supervision, and more medical services than are available in all but the best assisted living facilities today. The third level of care would be suitable for the most dependent older people, most of whom currently live in nursing homes, but some of whom are in assisted living facilities for the memory-impaired. This level would still provide resident-centered care and would feature a homier environment than exists in most nursing homes, but it would afford residents less privacy because privacy assumes less importance as people become increasingly dependent. Dignity and respect remain paramount, of course, but for the individual who is trapped in a body he cannot control, privacy sometimes turns into isolation, a lonely and frightening condition.

The view that assisted living and nursing home care should converge flies in the face of current conventional wisdom, which promotes further development of a "continuum of care." This continuum begins at home, with older people availing themselves of community services; it encompasses adult day care; it stretches to include assisted living; and ultimately it ends in the nursing home. But the fundamental principles of good assisted living apply equally to all long-term care, wherever it takes place. Assisted living, according to some of its most insightful proponents, is premised on a residential living environment that supports independence, on a philosophy that emphasizes choice and dignity, and on the capacity to provide services that meet individualized needs.[37] Quality in a nursing home can similarly be defined in terms of the physical environment, the social environment, and the adequacy of personal and medical assistance. There is no reason why assisted living communities and nursing homes, both forms of institutional long-term care—care administered once the individual has left her own home—should not be structured the same way, monitored and assessed the same way, and paid for the same way.

Assisted living is "the product of idealism, pragmatism, entrepreneurial impulse, and consumer hope."[38] If we build on that hope in the coming years, shoring it up with a long-term-care Medicare benefit, protecting it with suitable but not suffocating regulations, and nurturing it with innovations that derive from experience, then assisted living will become a boon for the baby boomers.

SEVEN

The Lure of Immortality

THE ULTIMATE way to ensure that the baby boomers won't have to worry about the perils of old age is to eradicate aging entirely. And that, according to a dozen or more biotechnology start-up companies with names like Elixir and Rejuvenon, is not entirely out of the question.[1] If the aging process could be stopped in its tracks, we would not need to think about dealing with frailty or to imagine designing better nursing homes or to ask whether assisted living is adequate for people with dementia. Nobody would develop age-associated diseases such as stroke or heart disease or Alzheimer's, nor would anyone have to face the assorted dependencies and disabilities that arise from weakened muscles, worn-down joints, and wobbly memories.

Scientists—and entrepreneurs—are increasingly thinking seriously about the possibility of abolishing or at least postponing aging. Philosophers and social scientists are beginning to consider the consequences of interfering with the aging process.[2] But as the twenty-first century begins, it is far from clear that the prevention of aging will be feasible, and even less clear that it would be a good idea if it were possible.

Ruth schatz became my patient on her 87th birthday. Her hazel eyes sparkled when she told me about her son: "A good boy, always telephones his mother, every day at eight o'clock. Rain or shine." Her eyes clouded over with tears when she spoke of her miscarriages, a story she had evidently repeated so many times that she had all the details down pat, even though everything else about the 1930s and 40s was distorted, like a reflection in rippling water. I think she said she had had three miscarriages, one when she was so far along in her pregnancy that the fetus she expelled—during a bloody sojourn in the bathroom after straining too hard—was fully formed. "Since then I've always taken milk of magnesia. Every night for the last sixty years. Thanks to the milk of magnesia, I carried all the way." She paused, trying hard to recall the birth of her miracle child, a story that sprouted from a kernel of truth but was greatly embellished by the time it emerged from her chapped lips. "The doctor said I would never be able to have children. That it was dangerous for me and that my womb would burst. So I took to bed after five months and stayed there for the rest of the time. I passed the eight-month mark. And then the ninth. And still he didn't come out. My Gerald wasn't born for ten months. He's a good boy," she began again. "He calls me every day at eight o'clock. Rain or shine."

Ruth was an attractive woman, although the sun had battered her fair skin over the years. She was a dermatologist's delight: she had monthly appointments during which the skin doctor assiduously inspected her for skin cancer, often finding a suspicious lesion on her face, her arms, or her chest, above the bathing suit line. She had actinic keratoses—benign, skin-induced areas of roughness and discoloration—and squamous cell carcinomas—superficial cancers that the dermatologist froze off or treated with topical medication. Ruth bragged when I first met her that she had had twenty-six spots removed, all of which were either malignant or pre-cancerous. Later she would tell me it was fifty, and once she reported, with complete seriousness, that it was five hundred.

Modern medicine had been good to Ruth. Not only had she outwitted the sun's determination to give her cancer, but she had also triumphed over the ravages of osteoarthritis. "My knees were very bad," she told me. "I kept house for my Edward—he was a good man. He never forgot my birthday. We were married for 55 years." As with the skin lesions, the numbers sometimes changed, and not always linearly with the passage of time. "Every year for my birthday he bought me something. Even during the Depression, when he had no job and no money, he gave me a box and he said, 'Ruth, you are the light of my life.' And inside I found earrings or a brooch or something else he could not afford." Sometimes after these digressions she remembered she had been explaining the origins of the wear-and-tear arthritis in her knees. "Every week, I got down on my knees and scrubbed the floor. And when I reached 70, my knees began to creak. They made a noise like this"—she made a clicking sound with her tongue that was meant to signify the noise of bone on bone. "And they hurt terribly. So I got new knees. First one, then the other. I used to have such pain when I walked. Now I can walk for miles." In addition to the new knees, Ruth had had a total hip replacement. She also had a pacemaker inserted after a small heart attack that was precipitated by her hip surgery. "I am a bionic woman," she told me proudly. "I will live forever."

The pacemaker had prevented fainting spells; the orthopedic surgery had maintained Ruth's mobility; the dermatologist's vigilance had kept her cancer-free. And there was more medical magic: cataract surgery preserved her vision; monthly B12 injections cured her anemia. But in her early eighties—her son Gerald could not pinpoint the exact year—Ruth became forgetful.

The changes were subtle at first. Instead of merely telling the same stories each time she met you, she related them two or even three times during a single encounter. Always an outstanding puzzle-solver, she could no longer figure out how to deal with novelty. If the street near her house was blocked off, she couldn't come up with an alternate route, even though she had lived in the same neighborhood for decades. Family relationships were particularly baffling to her. If you told her: "This is Joe's niece, Sylvia" and "Of course you remember Joe's sister, Eleanor," Ruth could not imagine that Eleanor might be Sylvia's mother. Numbers were perplexing as well. Ruth's concept of prices was rooted in the 1950s. The cashier at the local drugstore nearly called the police when she insisted that she would pay no more than a nickel for the newspaper, and only the intervention of another customer, who surreptitiously slipped the cashier another 45 cents, averted a showdown.

At first Gerald blamed his mother's behavior on his father's death. They had been interdependent for so long that she fell apart without him. Gerald brought his mother to a doctor, and for a while she took an antidepressant. But nothing slowed the relentless progression of her memory problems—not the antidepressant, not new glasses, not a hearing aid, not moving into senior housing where she had company and a weekly bingo game. Ruth, who had always been a reader, who always said that if she had been born twenty years later, she would have gone to college, was developing dementia.

Thanks to the lens implants and the joint replacements, she could see and she could walk, which compensated in part for her failing mind. But then she had another heart attack. It was a small one, but the cardiologists performed a special test that led them to conclude that Ruth was at risk of a fatal heart irregularity. "She's otherwise in good shape," the physician told her son. "The only thing that's likely to kill her is if she has a run of 'v tach' [ventricular tachycardia]. We can do something about that now. It's a pretty new approach, which involves replacing the old pacemaker with a combination pacemaker and implantable defibrillator. This not only detects an abnormally slow heartbeat, and kicks in with its own electrical signal; it can also tell if she goes into 'v tach' and will automatically deliver an electric shock to jolt her back to a normal rhythm. It's the same procedure we use during a cardiac arrest, but it's internal instead of external and it all happens automatically." The cardiologist beamed. "It's remarkable technology."

The cardiologist was right. It *is* remarkable technology, and there was nothing else besides the irregular heart rhythm that was likely to kill Ruth Schatz any time soon. With her brand-new implantable cardioverter defibrillator (ICD), Ruth lived another five years, becoming more and more demented with each birthday.

I knew the defibrillator was keeping Ruth alive because every few months it went off. She would scream—by itself, nothing unusual, since Ruth often screamed when she came across something unfamiliar or when she was lonely or inexplicably afraid. But the nurses at the nursing home—for by now Ruth needed the 24-hour care provided by a nursing home—learned to recognize the particularly anguished cries Ruth emitted when the device fired. "I've been shot!" she yelled sometimes. Or "I'm going to lose the baby!"[3]

The defibrillator protocol required that we send Ruth to the hospital whenever the device fired. So we dutifully called an ambulance and packed Ruth off to the nearest hospital, where she would be checked for evidence of a heart attack and for defibrillator malfunction. On her many trips, she never had either. But each time she went to the hospital, she was invariably sedated. It's not good for the other patients in a coronary care unit to have someone moan and shriek and claim that the nurses are all Nazis. When she returned to the nursing home, Ruth often remained sleepy and profoundly confused for days.

After the third visit to the hospital, Ruth's son called me up. "I know it's a little irregular," he said awkwardly. "I know the heart doctors say my mother should go to the hospital each time that, that—" he stuttered a little—"that blasted thing goes off. But what would be so bad about just letting her stay at the nursing home?" I agreed that his suggestion was entirely reasonable. The nursing staff were not convinced. They had protocols to follow, too, and they worried that they were not equipped to handle a patient who had just had a heart attack (if Ruth ever did have one) or whose defibrillator was going off when it shouldn't (in the event that ever happened). After a great deal of back-and-forth, the staff accepted the idea that Gerald was willing to take his chances. The defibrillator would be monitored, just as its pacemaker predecessor had been, at office visits using special machinery, but without hospitalization.

A few months later, Ruth began wailing for no discernible reason. I could not find a clear physical source of pain, but I prescribed analgesics anyway, just in case she was experiencing pain that she could not point to or describe. When Tylenol didn't work, I tried codeine, but that just made her hallucinate. She was convinced that birds were flying around her room and that if she went to sleep, they would peck her eyes out. She cried out that the "flapping" was terrible, and covered her ears. I stopped the codeine and the birds disappeared, but she continued to be intermittently paranoid. When the fire alarms went off, Ruth would call her son. She could no longer remember his phone number, but he had programmed the telephone so that she just had to press "1." She told him, panicked, "Gerald, there's a nuclear war!" She started saying "hoo, hoo, hoo" repeatedly, between mouthfuls at mealtimes, until the other residents demanded that she stay out of the dining room. Ruth was exiled to the hall outside her room.

Shortly after her 93rd birthday, the nursing home administrator transferred Ruth to another floor that seemed to Gerald more like a mental institution than a nursing home: residents roamed the halls in search of their long-dead mothers or the car keys they had been forced to surrender years ago. Ruth's hooting and wailing were drowned out by a dapper-looking elderly man who called out "come here, come here" whenever anything moved within his visual field, and by a very overweight woman who sang "Little Jack Horner" continuously.

It broke Gerald's heart to see his mother on the dementia unit. He made an appointment to meet with me and the facility social worker. I expected him to ask for another transfer, to a floor where the residents were quieter and less cognitively impaired. "It must be very hard for you to see your mother here," the social worker began tentatively.

Gerald surprised us by assuring us that it was difficult, but he knew it was where she belonged. He implored me to give her however much medication was necessary to calm her down. And then he asked whether there was any way to turn off the defibrillator.

For a moment, I was not sure I had understood him. Gerald had had a stroke, and his speech was a little slurred. Sometimes he had trouble finding the words to express himself.

He repeated his question, slowly and clearly, although this time it was a command. "I want you to turn the defibrillator off. If it weren't for that darned machine, my mother would be at peace now."

I had never had such a request. But patients and families routinely decided to forgo attempted cardiopulmonary resuscitation. The only way that Ruth could forgo CPR was to disable the implanted device. Moreover, withdrawal of medical therapy has long been ethically and legally acceptable when requested by a competent patient or her health care proxy.

I made sure that Gerald understood the implications. I particularly wanted him to realize that Ruth was not dependent on the defibrillator. She might well continue to live without it.

He understood. He just wanted it turned off.

I knew it could be done. I called up Ruth's cardiologist, who came over and had essentially the same conversation I had just had with Gerald. He tried to examine Ruth, who howled "ow ow ow" when he attempted to listen to her heart with his stethoscope. And then, very gently, he held a magnet over her chest, fiddled with a few dials, and the defibrillator was off.[4]

I prescribed medication for Ruth to control her agitation. Antipsychotics alone didn't work, nor did antidepressants, nor did anti-anxiety medication. It took a combination of medicines, in doses so high that Ruth slept much of the time, to soothe her nerves. She died in her sleep, three months to the day after the cardiologist turned off her defibrillator.

If this is what longer life is all about, most people want no part of it. Throughout recorded history, we find similar cautionary tales exhorting humankind to avoid the perils of eternal life. The ancient Greeks gave us the myth of Tithonus, a handsome young mortal who struck the fancy of Eos, goddess of the dawn. Eos, a strong-willed female, decided to marry Tithonus, but thought it a pity that he would not last very long, from her immortal perspective. She begged Zeus, the chief god, to confer immortality upon her beloved and, surprisingly, he obliged. But Eos forgot to request eternal youth along with eternal life, and after a few good years together, Tithonus began to age. He became increasingly debilitated, literally shriveled up, and ultimately was transformed into a grasshopper. Eos put him in a cage to chirp for all eternity.

In a strikingly similar, more contemporary tale, Jonathan Swift introduced us to the immortal Struldbruggs, encountered by Gulliver in his travels. These creatures age normally until they reach eighty. At that point, they are "not only opionative, peevish, covetous, morose, vain [and] talkative," but also incapable of friendship and affection. The least miserable of them are "those who turn to dotage and entirely lose their memories," since they at least are blissfully unaware of their state. Lest there be any doubt that immortality is a curse, Swift tells us that at ninety, "they lose their teeth and hair; they have at that age no distinction of taste, but eat and drink whatever they can get without relish or appetite . . . In talking, they forget the common appellation of things, and the names of persons, even of those who are their nearest friends and relations. For the same reason, they never can amuse themselves with reading, because their memory will not serve to carry them from the beginning of a sentence to the end, and by this defect, they are deprived of the only entertainment whereof they might otherwise be capable." Finally, the narrator relates that the Struldbruggs "were the most mortifying sight I ever beheld, and the women more horrible than the men. Besides the usual deformities of extreme old age, they acquired an additional ghastliness in proportion to their number of years, which is not to be described." He adds, in case the reader fails to grasp his message, that "my keen appetite for perpetuity of life was much abated" and regrets that sending a few Struldbruggs to his own country "to arm our people against the fear of death" would violate the country's laws.[5]

The risk that geriatric medicine might lengthen life without improving its quality is real. The debate about whether existing approaches to care will lead to "compression of morbidity" in which the period of disability and dependence shrinks while overall lifespan grows, or instead to increasingly long periods of frailty, is far from settled.[6] The rate of disability with old age has declined in recent years, giving greater credibility to the compression-of-morbidity proponents, but rates of *severe* disability remain unchanged. A few diehards argue that it is immaterial whether longer life comes at the price of disability; they balk at any attempt to suggest that adding "life to years" is more important than adding "years to life." All such decisions, they maintain, should be left to the individual. Some people, if they had the option, might conceivably choose to take a longevity pill—hoping, betting, or praying that they would not develop dementia or that scientists would soon find a way to reverse the currently permanent neurological damage caused by Alzheimer's disease. But unless treatment for dementia improves dramatically, the specter of robust bodies housing crumbling minds will continue to haunt us.

Tithonus, the Struldbruggs, and Ruth Schatz embody the dilemma of the current piecemeal strategy toward aging. Today's reality entails treating, and trying to cure, one disease at a time, which just props up failing bodies. Pro-longevists are fully cognizant of the limitations of this approach to aging. Proponents of a view known as the unitary theory of aging see Ruth Schatz (and others like her) as a dramatic illustration of why the right approach to controlling aging is to shut off the process altogether. This theory, which holds that there is an on/off switch, implies that finding this switch and learning how to control it will lead to the simultaneous preservation of the function of *all* bodily systems. The result, according to Richard Miller, a reputable pro-longevity scientist, will be an increase in the average lifespan to 112 years and in the maximum lifespan to 140 years.[7]

Scientists are hot on the trail of the switch. The most promising place to look for it is hidden among our genes. And the key may be in the lowly worm—in particular, a one-millimeter creature known as *Caenorhabditis elegans*, or *C. elegans* for short. It is technically a soil nematode, which means that it thrives on rotting vegetation. What has made *c. elegans* popular among biologists who study aging is that it is a multicellular organism and thus is a little more like people than is yeast, for example, whose longevity genes have also been studied. Moreover, this worm's body is transparent, allowing all 959 of its non-reproductive cells to be clearly visible under the microscope. *C. elegans* has a primitive nervous system and is capable of extremely rudimentary learning. It normally lives two to three weeks, which means experiments that involve genes affecting lifespan can be carried out in a reasonable period of time—unlike comparable experiments in rhesus monkeys, which live an average of 24 years.

Scientists at the biotechnology company Elixir, whose name is intended to invoke the elixir of life, have discovered that several distinct genes affect longevity in *C. elegans*. Mutations at a single point in the gene can double the worm's average lifespan, and mutations in two different longevity genes can nearly triple its lifespan. What's more, the worm's longevity-controlling genes are almost identical to those found in fruit flies, yeast, and mice, raising the possibility that these genes represent a universal control mechanism for life expectancy. As the Elixir founding scientists put it, "When single genes are changed, animals that should be old stay young. In humans, these mutants would be analogous to a ninety-year-old who looks and feels forty-five. On this basis, we begin to think of aging as a disease that can be cured, or at least postponed. This paradigm shift is due largely to the analysis of single-gene mutations that influence aging in model organisms."[8]

Identifying the genes associated with aging will not immediately lead to a way to turn them off, however. Scientists figured out the chemical structure of hemoglobin in 1956, subsequently deduced the sequence of the gene for this protein in 1978, and from that information arrived at an understanding of how an abnormal form of the protein causes the malformation of red blood cells that produce the disease sickle cell anemia.[9] But nearly three decades later, there is still no cure for sickle cell anemia. The cystic fibrosis story is similar. Cystic fibrosis, the most common autosomal recessive disease in the western hemisphere, is another genetic disease that involves the mutation of a single gene. This gene is responsible for producing a substance necessary to keep the lungs from clogging up with secretions. In 1985 a mutation was pinpointed to a small region of chromosome 7, and in 1989 the defective gene responsible for cystic fibrosis was isolated. Although these discoveries led to enormous progress in the understanding of cystic fibrosis, and even to partially successful gene therapy, there is still no cure for the disease.

Even if we could cure these genetic diseases, we would not necessarily be able to prevent aging. Curing sickle cell anemia or cystic fibrosis through genetic techniques would involve repairing or replacing the abnormal gene, whereas delaying aging would entail turning off the gene. Many facets of gene regulation are unclear—just how it works, why genes sometimes make proteins and sometimes do not, and why genes sometimes make a great deal of protein and sometimes only a little.

It is possible that scientists will discover indirect ways of influencing the switch, even if they can't figure out precisely how to turn it off. One possible strategy, in vogue in the 1990s, is to manipulate telomeres. All chromosomes have mysterious repeating sequences of DNA at their tips, known as telomeres. As cells divide and age, the telomeres become shorter and shorter until, at some critical length, the cells can no longer divide. The enzyme telomerase prevents telomeres from shortening, in principle conferring immortality on cells. And in fact, large quantities of telomerase are present in cancerous cells, allowing them to multiply indefinitely. Michael West, a colorful, charismatic, and controversial scientist, was one of the early believers in telomeres as the key to aging.[10] West—erstwhile fundamentalist Christian born again as a physician and then anew as a molecular biologist—started a company he called Geron to isolate the gene for telomerase. The gene was found and sequenced by scientists under contract to Geron, but the leap from a DNA sequence to a pill for immortality has proved at least as great as the leap from *C. elegans* to human beings. West himself has moved on to other strategies for life extension, principally centered on therapeutic cloning, or the use of stem cells to make new body parts to replace worn-out old ones. He continues to believe that death is the enemy, commenting that "the life cycle [is] completely unacceptable."[11]

The most theoretically plausible avenue to preventing or delaying aging, given the contemporary state of knowledge, is caloric restriction. In rodents, at least, consumption of only 60 percent of the usual caloric intake—while maintaining a balanced diet, which is no mean feat—leads to a 30 percent increase in lifespan. No one has proved that the phenomenon holds in primates, since the experiments on calorically restricted monkeys have not been going on long enough to permit conclusions about longevity. The emaciated monkeys do show indirect evidence that they are aging slowly: their immune systems are more vigilant, for example, than those of their chunkier peers. But without any good markers for aging—and there aren't any at present—the only way to decide if aging has been delayed is to wait and see how long it takes before the monkeys die.

Few scientists believe that draconian restrictions on eating would be tolerable to very many people, even with life extension as a potent motivator. Approximately 30 percent of the American population is currently thought to be obese.[12] Even claims that their eating habits are shortening their lives have been insufficient to induce these overweight individuals to eat less and exercise more, the only certain means to weight loss. The scientist's dream is therefore not to discover a means of changing behavior but rather to find a chemical compound that mimics the biochemical effects of caloric restriction. The idea is to trick the body into thinking it is starving and inducing it to go into self-preservation mode. Just as people learn to be frugal when economic conditions are poor, organisms likewise shift to a low metabolic state when the food supply is meager. Once resources become plentiful, creatures can again afford to maintain their bodies and to reproduce. But when food is limited, the balance between self-maintenance and procreation switches to the most basic cellular upkeep and repair. So far, substances that looked as if they might be "caloric restriction mimetics" such as 2DG (2-deoxy-D-glucose), which disrupts glucose metabolism in rats, turned out to be toxic when given in high enough doses or over long enough time periods to potentially affect aging.[13] The search for the holy grail continues.

If longevity genes, telomerase research, and caloric restriction are not about to lead to an anti-aging pill anytime soon, perhaps antioxidants will be the answer. Much of the damage to cells and to genetic material, damage that produces aging by increasing the organism's vulnerability to disease, may be caused by free radicals. Since these chemically highly active molecules are the by-product of normal metabolism, the body has already evolved other chemicals that mop up free radicals. Theoretically, these naturally occurring clean-up agents may retard aging. A variety of compounds fit the bill, including superoxide dismutase and vitamin E. Antioxidants may yet prove to play a role in delaying aging, since one of the consequences of caloric restriction, which does delay aging at least in mice, is less metabolic activity and less free radical production. But for the present, there are no certain pathways to the fountain of youth.

If scientists do produce an anti-aging potion, we will still not be immortal. Even if there is a switch that sets aging in motion, turning off the switch will not lead to indefinite prolongation of life. In the absence of systems for repair, organs will ultimately weaken and fail. And the body does not have any way of achieving continual repair. Aging occurs because natural selection favored people who survived long enough to reproduce, but it had no way of promoting longevity after the reproductive years are over. The reason, for example, why women do not die at menopause (or, perhaps more plausibly, fifteen years after menopause when they have launched their last child into some semblance of self-sufficiency) is that engineering a person to survive long enough to reproduce requires building in redundancy. The odds of living to about age 55 are good only if the body has considerable reserves. It is that excess capacity, that cushion allowing survival despite famine and floods, which permits us to age at all. And of course finding the gene that controls longevity would not eliminate our capacity for violence or the possibility of accidental death. In any event, for the baby boomers, many of whom are already on the cusp of old age, life extension is not in the cards.

Figuring out how to live to age 140 may not be imminent, but we do have in our midst today some examples of people who live to a ripe old age with hardly any medical problems and very little disability. Centenarians, of whom there were slightly over 88,000 in the United States in the year 2004, come close to the pro-longevist ideal and might provide valuable clues to successful aging.[14]

Tom Perls, a geriatrician and founder of the New England Centenarian Study, agrees. He discovered that centenarians are often healthier and more vigorous than their octogenarian counterparts; that they are likely to have nonagenarian siblings; and that they also looked younger and more vigorous than their peers when they were 70, 50, and even 30 years old. They have typically escaped catastrophic illnesses throughout their lives, and they have frequently evaded many, if not all, the diseases commonly associated with aging, including heart disease and dementia. They have managed the feat of "successful aging," not only remaining disease-free until the end but also maintaining a high level of mental and physical functioning and staying actively engaged with life.[15]

The poster child of centenarians was Jeanne Calment, a French woman who upon her death at the age of 122 was the oldest documented human being in history. She celebrated each birthday with reporters, beginning at age 115. Nearly blind and very hard of hearing, she remained intellectually intact until her last years, when she lost a little of her sparkle. She smoked until she was 110, to the dismay of healthy life-style gurus, but in partial compensation she rode a bicycle until she turned 100. When asked what accounted for her longevity—as though the secret could be discerned by mere introspection—she attributed her long life to her sense of humor.[16]

Equally famous are the long-lived Okinawans.[17] Their life expectancy is the greatest in the world, exceeding that of their relatively long-lived neighbors in mainland Japan. A baby girl born in Okinawa today can expect to live to age 86. Okinawa has the highest rate of centenarians of any country, currently 34/100,000, compared with only 10/100,000 in the United States. Okinawans have far lower rates of heart disease, stroke, and cancer than do their counterparts in the western world. Part of their success probably comes from their diet—they eat primarily grains, fruits, and vegetables, with fish rather than meat as a major protein source. And they take in fewer calories, on average 500 fewer per day, than Americans. They also live in a warm, sunny climate; they have high rates of job satisfaction; and their society is known for its excellent social networks and support systems. Most likely, however, a large part of their propensity toward long life is genetic. A fairly homogeneous population, they have only recently begun to abandon their traditional villages and leave the beautiful island that is attracting increasing attention from the outside world.

Centenarians have something important to teach. Often they have wisdom arising from their accumulated experiences which they enjoy sharing, and which they are able to share because they are not burdened by multiple maladies, each with its own demanding regimen of pills, monitoring tests, and physician visits. Their world is the antithesis of the elderly community in Florida, which has developed a culture that revolves around their health. The average elderly Floridian sees multiple specialists, often making more than one physician visit each week. Gathered around the table while eating an "early bird special," they exchange doctor stories. When one member of the group reports that he has seen a new specialist—perhaps a rheumatologist has joined the ranks of his cardiologist, urologist, and general internist—the others eagerly add the new doctor to their own lists of "providers."[18] In parts of Florida, the state with the largest elderly contingent in the United States, Medicare spends more than twice as much per capita for health care as it does anywhere else. What its citizens get in exchange for this largesse is more hospital days, more tests, more ICU admissions, and more subspecialty consultations in the last six months of life, with no evidence that the additional attention improves the quality of care.[19]

Centenarians have another lesson for us as well. The usual claim is that centenarians remain robust until a catastrophic event occurs, at which time, like the "one-hoss shay" of Oliver Wendell Holmes, they collapse completely.[20] Centenarians are different from other people in that the aging process has been postponed—at age 95, their organs are like those of a typical 75-year-old. But there is no reason to believe that their organs are programmed to fail simultaneously. The reason the centenarian dies from his pneumonia or his heart attack is that doctors do not aggressively treat their 100-plus-year-old patients—they do not routinely admit them to the intensive care unit, place them on a breathing machine, start dialysis, or initiate any of the other interventions that are commonplace in octogenarians. Centenarians die quickly because we let them, and 85-year-olds die slowly because we don't.[21]

THOUGH not strictly speaking a centenarian—he was only 99—Bob Murdoch had all the hallmarks of a man who has aged successfully. He lived in a nursing home, but only because his wife had needed nursing home care. He had wanted to be with her, and at the time when he moved in, the admissions requirements were less stringent than they are today. Bob had been totally devoted to his ailing wife, who was blind, demented, and had breast cancer. He helped her wash up and get dressed, he went to concerts with her, and he talked to her. They played bingo as a duo, each compensating for the other's weakness—she could not see, he could scarcely hear. Above all, when she started to lose interest in the world around her, when she began spending most of her days sitting quietly in a chair, he sat beside her, holding her hand. When Gertrude died, Bob was devastated. He acknowledged that he had lost his reason for living. He said he wanted to die. But he was only 95, and it wasn't yet his time.

After a six-month mourning period, buoyed up by his religious faith, encouraged by visits from his priest and a few loyal cousins—he had no children—Bob began to regain his former vitality. He resumed going out to lunch with the other men on his floor; he joined an exercise group; he subscribed to and read the newspaper each day. Apart from his difficulty in hearing and some arthritis, Bob had no medical problems.

His 98th year was a bit trying. He managed to fracture both his ankle and his hip before I realized that he did have one significant medical condition—osteoporosis. We tend to think of osteoporosis as a disease of postmenopausal women, and to a large extent it is, but men are not immune; they just tend to be older than their female counterparts when they get it. If they make it into their nineties, their risk is considerable. By age 90, a third of all women and one-sixth of men will have fractured a hip.[22]

Bob's recovery from his fractures was quick and uneventful. However, he developed intolerable side effects from the bone-strengthening medicine I prescribed, and only with a fair amount of arm-twisting would he agree to stay on calcium and vitamin D supplements. "I don't like pills," he told me. But he went along with the recommendations of his physical therapist and emerged unscathed from his encounters with orthopedists. Unlike many old people who break their bones, he was left without disabilities. He did not even need a cane.

Shortly after his 99th birthday, Bob came down with a respiratory infection. It was flu season, and there was an outbreak in the nursing home. He had had a flu shot, but his immune system was not what it had once been, and he probably had been unable to make the antibodies against the influenza virus that the flu shot was meant to stimulate.

He was mildly feverish for a day, and then, precipitously, he became extremely ill. His temperature soared, his breathing became labored, he had no appetite. A hurried consultation with his family—the faithful cousins—produced a consensus that Bob should be treated at the nursing home and not rushed off to the hospital. When he was becoming dehydrated from not drinking enough as his fever raged, another conversation led to the decision to forgo intravenous fluids. He would be offered his favorite juices and would be given antibiotics if he was alert enough to take the pills, but we would not try any "heroics." And heroics, to Bob Murdoch, meant hospitals and intravenous drips as well as breathing machines.

A day later, Bob lapsed into unconsciousness. He could no longer take anything by mouth. He was very congested and was struggling to breathe, so I ordered oxygen and respiratory treatments administered through a nebulizer. That helped a little, but he still appeared uncomfortable. His lips turned blue, and the device we slipped onto his finger to measure the amount of oxygen in his system confirmed that his lungs were failing. I ordered small doses of morphine, which immediately eased his breathing. His nursing assistant, who had known him for years and affectionately called him grandpa, put cool washcloths on his face since even round-the-clock acetaminophen suppositories did not bring his temperature down. Bob Murdoch never woke up. A mere three days after he came down with a sore throat, muscle aches, and fever, he was dead.

Did Bob die because of multiple complications of the flu? There was no evidence that he had had a heart attack, a common cause of the excess mortality attributed to influenza. Among older people with weak hearts, the added strain of fighting an infection can be too much, and they go into heart failure or have a heart attack. Bob's electrocardiogram remained normal, however, except for showing that his heart had sped up, as typically happens with fever. He did not have the telltale rales of heart failure on physical examination. A chest X-ray, taken at the onset of his sickness, showed no evidence of the fluid that accumulates in the lungs when the heart does not pump sufficiently vigorously. Did his kidneys shut down, precipitating the end? He continued to urinate until he had stopped drinking entirely, and his blood tests when he first became ill indicated that his kidneys were working well.

Would Bob Murdoch have survived if he had gone to the hospital and received aggressive treatment? He might have. But to his friends and relatives, to the nurse taking care of him, and to me, his fulminant illness was clearly a turning point. Too often, we had seen elderly patients rushed to the hospital, rescued from the brink of death, and returned to a far lower level of functioning than they had previously enjoyed. Not only that, but within months the cycle was repeated, each rescue leaving these patients weaker and more debilitated. Finally—weeks, months, or occasionally years later—they succumbed despite the physician's best efforts. Bob's message, and perhaps that of most centenarians, is that there comes a time to stop.

SUCCESSFUL life extension—that is, doing more than eliminating premature death and instead increasing both average and maximal lifespan—would create a slew of social problems. Overpopulation is an issue in much of the world, and without dramatic declines in fertility in the Third World, a marked decrease in the death rate would further exacerbate the problem. In the developed world, where life expectancy already far exceeds that of the Third World, the birth rate has in fact plummeted—in some countries, such as Germany and Italy, falling below replacement levels.[23] What this means, if the trend continues as age at death rises, is that the age distribution in societies characterized by extreme longevity will shift so that there are hardly any young people at all. For a country like Germany, with a fertility rate of 1.38 children born per woman, even without any increase in lifespan the population pyramid is expected to turn into a virtual rectangle by 2050; almost the same number of people will be in every age bracket from infancy to age 85. If the average lifespan increases markedly, the number of old people could exceed the number of younger individuals. In the United States, the old age dependency ratio, or the ratio of the population over 65 to the population between ages 20 and 64 who will support them (assuming that the new crop of 90- and 100-year-olds will not be holding down paying jobs), may rise to 56/100 in the year 2075.[24] This implies that every couple, both members of whom are employed, will need to support (in addition to their children) one older person.

A topsy-turvy age pyramid will require a major change in the allocation of resources. In the 2005 fiscal year, the United States spent a net $295 billion on Medicare. Although Medicare insures both the elderly and the disabled, 85 percent of the enrollees are the over-65 group, accounting for the lion's share of the expenditures. Moreover, fully a third of the Medicaid budget goes to long-term care for the elderly. While the medical costs for older people would presumably go down if there were a new, exceptionally vigorous breed who remained healthy until, abruptly, all their organ systems failed, their overall resource use would still rise because of their sheer numbers and their economic dependency.

Extending life will create grave injustice if it is not equally available to all citizens. If achieving longevity turns out to involve yearly, or for that matter monthly, infusions of stem cells or some similar technological fix, the costs associated with the procedure could be extraordinary. Assuming this intervention will not be covered by medical insurance, just as other "enhancements" such as liposuction or Botox injections or growth hormone shots are not, then living to age 112 would effectively be available only to the rich.[25] The gap between the haves and have-nots, which has been increasing over the last decade in the United States, would be greatly magnified. From an international perspective, the disparities between countries would also multiply, as the gap in life expectancy between the richest and the poorest countries would grow from the current shocking 43 years (life expectancy at birth is 37.4 years in Angola versus 80.6 years in Japan) to a mind-boggling 75 years.[26] The hatred between societies, rooted to some extent in jealousy, could intensify further.

Whether individuals would really want to live to age 110 or 140 is far from clear. Philosophers refer to those who accept the inevitability of human mortality, and a species-specific upper bound on lifespan, as "apologists."[27] The acceptance of the cycle of human life, with its characteristic renewal as well as decay, is seen by some as at best perverse romanticism and at worst unimaginative anachronism. But is the statement that living things are born, grow, and die really value-laden, or is it simply an eternal truth? And if it is an acknowledgment of a pervasive reality, perhaps it is not a manifestation of a stunted imagination to suggest that the cycle of life, far from being arbitrary and susceptible to scientific manipulation, is one of the few quintessential features of existence. The President's Council on Bioethics, in its report on biotechnology and the pursuit of happiness, discusses the pros and cons of agelessness. The authors view the quest for ever-greater longevity as a manifestation of narcissism, arguing instead that "generation and nurture, dependency and reciprocated generosity, are in some harmony of proportion, and there is a pace of journey, a coordinated coherence of meter and rhyme within the repeated cycles of birth, ascendancy, and decline—a balance and beauty of love and renewal giving answer to death that, however poignant, bespeaks the possibility of meaning and goodness in the human experience. All this might be overthrown or forgotten in the rush to fashion a technological project only along the gradient of our open-ended desires and ambitions."[28]

Clearly, certain aspects of the human life course can be changed and in fact have been changed. In 1900, 30 percent of all deaths occurred in children under five years of age.[29] Today, babies die prematurely primarily if they are born with a defect, typically involving the heart or brain, and small numbers of young children die of injuries or cancer. As a result, only 1.4 percent of all deaths occur in children under the age of five.[30] The claim that the cycle of birth, maturation, old age, and death is *natural* does not rest on the assumption that it has been historically invariant. Moreover, the changed expectations about longevity have had profound social ramifications. Couples once had many children —not just because of a lack of birth control, but also because childhood mortality rates were so high that a large number of births were needed to be sure that at least one offspring would survive to farm the land. The relative rarity of old people won them awe and respect in early America; the presumption was that they must have done something right to deserve their longevity. This was consistent with the ideas of the Puritans, who believed that everything existed for a purpose, and thus survival to old age was a sign of God's purpose. As the numbers of old people grew in America and they became an increasing economic burden on the young, they ceased to be venerated.[31] Contributing also to the shift in attitudes was the broader egalitarian revolution between 1770 and 1820 that changed relations between classes, races, and sexes, as well as between the generations.[32] But despite the changes brought about by improvements in health and sanitation, finitude has remained a defining condition of human existence.

The cycle of life is all around us—in the seasons, in the plants and animals that share our planet. We capture the eternal circle in our civil institutions, whether in the calendar, with its yearly repetition of holidays, or in the rites of passage characteristic of every culture. We have marriage ceremonies and funerals; we have graduations to mark the completion of a course of schooling. It is no coincidence that one of the most famous biblical passages is from Ecclesiastes:

> One generation goes, another comes,
> But the earth remains the same forever.
> The sun rises, and the sun sets—
> And glides back to where it rises.

And later, Ecclesiastes continues:

> A season is set for everything, a time for
>   every experience under heaven:
> A time for being born and a time for dying,
> A time for planting and a time for uprooting the planted;
> A time for slaying and a time for healing,
> A time for tearing down and a time for building up,
> A time for weeping and a time for laughing,
> A time for wailing and a time for dancing . . .[33]

The knowledge of our own mortality has shaped human culture. There have always been fringe efforts to defy death, from Ponce de León's search for the Fountain of Youth in the swamps of Florida to Elie Metchnikoff's self-administered injections of ground animal testicles.[34] But the traditional human response to the all too painful awareness of our transience has been to embark on "immortality projects." Ernest Becker invented the phrase, reflecting his view that finitude is the fundamental determinant of human psychology.[35] A healthy response to our unique ability to understand our future is to immortalize ourselves through our creations. The most concrete creation is our children—they carry our genes, they bear the imprint of their upbringing, they are the most universally available vessels of immortality. The reason infertility is so traumatic for many couples, and childlessness such a disappointment to many who never find a partner, is not just that bringing up children is rewarding, but that the failure to have offspring can have profound emotional consequences.

Immortality projects can take many different forms. Works of art, music, and literature are examples—they serve as legacies to subsequent generations. We feel pain and a profound sense of loss when cherished antiquities are destroyed because we recognize intuitively that they represent a link to the past, that they are the tangible embodiment of our ancestors.

Executives and entrepreneurs likewise are in the business of creating immortality projects. Founding a company—nurturing it, seeing it grow—is a source of more than monetary satisfaction. Inventors create devices, scientists undertake research, mathematicians prove theorems, all of which allow them to live on after their earthly death. The projects do not need to be as grandiose or as concrete as erecting a building or writing a book, however. The athletic coach who molds a team is engaged in creation, as is a teacher who prepares her students to face the world. The nurse who touches hundreds, perhaps thousands, with her caring and her competence has a diffuse but equally real claim on immortality.

I am not arguing that if people were immortal or even if they lived to 150, they would, paradoxically, accomplish less than they do now—although the conservative philosopher Leon Kass, the chair of President George W. Bush's Bioethics Council, has made exactly that claim. Kass argues that finitude is good for us, in large measure because "to know and to feel that one goes around only once, and that the deadline is not out of sight, is for many people the necessary spur to the pursuit of something worthwhile. . . . Mortality makes life matter."[36] I am convinced that despite greater longevity people would still be driven to create a legacy, though they might procrastinate, confident that they had plenty of time remaining, and ultimately never achieve anything noteworthy. My contention is not that it is good to be mortal because it promotes productivity, but rather that mortality is simply a reality. The time-honored human coping mechanism, over and beyond phantasmagorical dreams of perpetual life, is the immortality project. These efforts are the ultimate form of sublimation, of transforming our painful awareness of our own limits into enduring memories. They are the way we leave a mark on the world, even after we ourselves have departed.

EIGHT

Making the Most of the Retirement Years

WHETHER we live to be 150 or must reconcile ourselves to the more modest but already commonplace endpoint of 85 years, we are experiencing unprecedented longevity. Greater longevity means that we have to figure out how to spend twenty or more years of retirement. Just as we need to determine how best to address our health needs as we age, and to come up with good solutions for where we live, so too we have to consider what we will spend our time doing.

If we look to organizations such as the American Association of Retired Persons (AARP) for advice about what to do with all those extra years, we are apt to be told that retirement is a kind of extended vacation. And indeed, increasing numbers of older people are taking the trip they always wanted to take, whether it's the low-budget Elderhostel variety or the more upscale Alaskan cruise or European jaunt. But while travel is enjoyable for affluent and robust retirees, it isn't feasible for more debilitated elders, and it's seldom a full-time occupation for anyone.

Retirement magazines such as AARP's advertise a variety of other pastimes, from playing golf to going to the theater. But as with travel, these activities are based on a view of old age as a time for recreation. Having fun is fine if it's a reward for hard work or a diversion from something else, but most people are not satisfied with nonstop entertainment. The idea that older people have contributed enough and should be on the receiving end, that it's fine to stop giving and time to start taking, is like advocating an all-dessert diet. Perhaps older people should not be required to eat spinach if they don't care for it, or perhaps they should be encouraged to stop eating it Popeye-style, straight out of the can, and instead learn to make an elegant soufflé. But abandoning vegetables entirely is not a viable option for older people any more than it is for their younger counterparts.

Twenty years is a long time for continuous vacation. The baby boomers are going to want something more. The leisure theory of retirement, embodied in sterile, artificial retirement communities such as the original Sun City, will not do. We tend to think instead that old age should be a time of self-fulfillment. Unconstrained by family responsibilities and the need to earn a livelihood, the good life in old age is assumed to entail independence and personal gratification. But many older people are discovering that what gives meaning to their lives is not the pursuit of pleasure, but rather membership in a larger community. Giving to others is proving to be the ultimate source of self-fulfillment.

Since she had only embarked on her professional career at the age of 53, my mother was hardly about to call it quits at age 65.

For a few precious years, she had devoted herself to her clients, serving as a psychiatric social worker. She loved her work and planned to continue as long as possible.

Ilse started going to school after I graduated from college. Throughout my undergraduate years she had looked enviously at the books I brought home, marveling at the stories I told of inspiring lecturers and stimulating class discussions. She had never gone to college. She had not even gone to high school. Her formal education had stopped abruptly when she was 13 years old.

Actually, her schooling had begun to fizzle out even earlier, when she was expelled from school because Jews were no longer allowed to attend German public schools. Ilse lived in Stettin, a medium-sized port city on the Oder River in Nazi Germany. She transferred to a Jewish school, but within a few months, many of her teachers were arrested and taken away, never to be seen again. When she turned 13, her parents concluded they could not remain in Germany any longer. They arranged to travel to Shanghai, China, one of the only countries in the world to which German Jews could immigrate in 1939. But they thought their daughter would fare better in Europe under the protection of the Red Cross, an option for a few thousand children who left Germany on one of the "Kindertransports." Most went to England. Ilse was one of several hundred children who went to Belgium.

In Belgium she lived in a "children's home," which was essentially an orphanage. She was treated as though she had always been poor, did not have parents, and was devoid of manners, culture, or education. In fact, she had lived in a conventional middle-class household, with two respectable parents, and had always been a good student. But she did not know French. Until she mastered French, further schooling was out of the question.

Before Ilse and the other refugees had a chance to learn much French, the Nazis invaded Belgium. The group of one hundred, who ranged in age from 2 to 19, were taken in boxcars to a new destination in southern France. They would spend the next four years hiding out in France, first in a vermin-infested barn, then in a dilapidated castle. Starved for books, Ilse read and reread the handful of novels that somehow made their way into the group's possession. She read James Fenimore Cooper's *The Last of the Mohicans* in French, at least three times. Ditto for *Germinal* by Émile Zola. But she had no regular instruction in anything other than the art of survival.

The prospects for making it to the end of the war were dim, much less the chance of going to school and leading any semblance of a normal adolescence. At one point in 1942, the older teenagers were rounded up by the Vichy police and brought to Vernet, which was euphemistically known as a "transit camp." It was in fact a French concentration camp, from which those who survived the meager rations and ill treatment were sent by train to death camps in Poland. Miraculously, the forty children from the Castle of La Hille who were "interned" at Vernet were released—thanks to the bluff of their director, who had the audacity to storm into the camp and stay there until her charges were allowed to go. She insisted the children were under the protection of the Swiss Red Cross and that the police would get in trouble if they were harmed. The children *were* under the protection of the Red Cross, but it was unlikely that the Swiss would have intervened on their behalf, and even less likely that the Swiss could or would have caused trouble for the French. But evidently the French officials felt that dealing with the agitator in their midst was more trouble than it was worth, and they decided to send the children back to the castle in southern France instead of to Auschwitz.

Ilse and the other teens who had been rescued from the brink of death concluded they were no longer safe in France. In small groups, they attempted to cross the border into Switzerland. Most of them made it. A few were captured by the Swiss border guards and turned over to the Gestapo.[1] Ilse was one of the lucky ones.

The Swiss offered neither education nor jobs to the few refugees to whom they reluctantly provided shelter. The exception was in nursing: the Swiss needed nurses, so they allowed foreigners to take a few classes, obtaining roughly the equivalent of a practical nursing degree. Ilse spent the remainder of the war working in Geneva, typically 12-hour shifts, six days a week. She never saw her parents again; they both died in Shanghai.

In 1945, Ilse managed to contact friends of her parents who lived in New York City and received an affidavit to immigrate to the United States. On the basis of her experience as a "baby nurse" in Switzerland, she found a position as a nanny and later as a nursery school teacher. She married, gave birth to me, and continued working. She was fluent in three languages and dreamed of becoming a translator at the United Nations. But you couldn't become an interpreter without a college degree; and you couldn't enter college without a high school diploma. Ilse didn't have one, and she couldn't imagine taking the tests in algebra, geometry, and science that would be required to obtain a diploma.

Then, in the 1970s, New York University established its "University Without Walls" program. NYU made two promises: students could receive credit for "life experiences," and they would be accepted into a degree program without high school equivalency tests if they enrolled in—and completed the requirements for—two college-level courses. Ilse had ample life experiences, and I helped her argue that her success as a preschool teacher presupposed a knowledge of early childhood psychology. She enrolled in a literature class and a psychology course and passed both easily. She was on her way to becoming a college graduate.

College courses were exciting, but to fulfill her dream of becoming a social worker, Ilse had to attend graduate school. She was accepted at the Wurzweiler School of Social Work of Yeshiva University in 1976; at age 53 she was awarded the coveted Master of Social Work degree.

My mother was a natural. She decided to switch from working with small children to caring for older adults, embarking on a career in providing psychotherapy. She saw her clients in the office and sometimes in their homes. They loved her. Her boss recognized that she was a jewel. And she thrived on the work. Reaching the age at which she became eligible for Social Security was hardly a reason to stop.

Ilse wasn't compelled to work to support herself—her husband had a good job, so her decision to work was based on a personal assessment of its value. Over time, she decided she would prefer to continue on a part-time basis. She found she was able to develop relationships with people whom the psychiatrists had long ago dismissed as too schizoid to be able to form relationships at all. Her quiet style, her unthreatening manner, and her perseverance led the most recalcitrant patients to open up to her. But she didn't want to spend all her time with psychiatric patients. There were too many other interesting possibilities in the world.

Ilse traveled and eventually moved to the Boston area to spend time with her grandchildren. When my oldest son was in high school, he often had lunch with her, telling her about the pains and frustrations of adolescence. She was well-suited to be his confidante—family, but not a parent, non-judgmental, a good listener. She was delighted to spend time with this thoughtful, intelligent young man who was struggling to figure out who he was and what he wanted from life. At his age, she hadn't known if she would have a life at all.

When Ilse turned 70, she decided to cut back her social work practice further. She liked the freedom to set her own hours and to go away for extended periods. But she also wanted new challenges—to use her skills in new ways. She decided to volunteer as a tutor at her local public library and was assigned to a young Chinese woman who knew no English. Ilse remembered all too well arriving in New York, fluent in French and German, with a smattering of Hebrew, but unable to understand a word of English. She wished she had had a private tutor to speak with her, to suggest books for her to read, and simply to encourage her. Her student adored her: she felt so safe with Ilse that for a while she refused to join a conversation group with other emigrants like herself. In exchange for her English lessons, she took Ilse to Chinatown and introduced her to genuine Chinese cooking.

Tutoring a single student was not enough for Ilse. She volunteered to be a "book lady" for the library, driving around town delivering books to shut-ins. She also volunteered at a nearby nursing home, providing psychotherapy to residents who had refused to see a psychiatrist but who opened up like roses on a sunny day when Ilse came to talk to them.

At age 79, nearly 80, my mother is still going strong. She takes brisk walks every day, rain or shine. She reads books in French and German just to make sure she doesn't forget those languages. Mainly she wants to remain engaged with the world. She wants to keep on doing things for other people, seizing whatever opportunities come her way. I think her motto is "help till you yelp."

Older people do not always feel the need to cut back or to try something different just because they have reached the age of 65—or even 70 or 80, though they are in the minority if they don't: only 8 percent of those over 75 work.[2] These vigorous seniors do not need new kinds of work or new types of relationships to feel valued. They have the stamina and the health and the interest to keep on doing what they have always done.

Bill and Reuben (Ruby) Landau are law partners who continue to ply their trade at ages 73 and 100, respectively. Reuben founded the firm of Landau and Landau in the 1920s. At one time, the corporate practice boasted ten lawyers. Now it's down to two: father and son. Both are remarkably healthy, physically and mentally. Bill told a *New York Times* reporter writing a story on centenarians that he sometimes dreamed of quitting the practice and spending his time playing tennis in Florida or perfecting the magic show he occasionally performs for charities. But when he suggested retiring, he commented, his father complained, "What would I doooooo?" "Just like that. 'Doooooo,'" Bill lamented.

"How do you say no to a 100-year-old man? You can't. I can't. I can't be that selfish. Besides, he'd disown me." So Ruby continued to walk every morning from his home in Cambridge to his office in downtown Boston, an hour each way, until the partners decided that Ruby's living room had it all over the city.[3]

One of my personal heroes is Daniel Schorr, another remarkable exemplar of the tradition of keep-on-doing-what-you've-always-done. At age 89, he continues to serve as Senior News Analyst for National Public Radio (NPR), appearing regularly on *All Things Considered* and *Weekend Edition*, where he delivers pungent and insightful commentary on the news. A journalist since serving in the U.S. Army Intelligence during World War II, he has had a distinguished, varied, and at times tendentious career. He began by writing from Western Europe for the *Christian Science Monitor* and then moved to the *New York Times*, for whom he reported on the rebirth of postwar Europe. In 1953 he joined CBS News as its diplomatic correspondent in Washington and then opened a CBS bureau in Moscow, where he finagled an exclusive television interview with Nikita Khrushchev. His interview did not endear him to the Soviet regime, leading him to move to a new post in Washington.

Schorr managed to be in many of the world's hot spots and became the CBS Bureau Chief for Germany and Eastern Europe just in time to cover the building of the Berlin Wall. He returned to Washington in 1966, which positioned him perfectly to serve as the chief Watergate correspondent for CBS when that scandal broke in 1972. Schorr ran into trouble for his insistence that he would not betray a source and left CBS after narrowly avoiding a contempt citation by the House Ethics Committee. He then spent several years as a professor of journalism at the University of California in Berkeley, but found the academic life too tame. He plunged back into the thick of things by helping to found CNN (1979) and serving as its senior correspondent. At age 69, he left CNN in a dispute over an effort to limit his editorial independence and has spent what would conventionally be the retirement years as a crusty correspondent for NPR.[4]

A minority of older people take up an entirely new career after they retire from their midlife work. Betty Friedan's book *The Fountain of Age* is replete with examples of older women (though more often the 65- to 70-year-olds than the 80- to 85-year-olds) finding new sources of passionate engagement.[5] Sometimes these are longstanding hobbies to which they can now devote more time. Occasionally they discover new talents, following in the footsteps of Grandma Moses.

Grandma Moses was born Anna Mary Robertson in 1860 on a farm in Greenwich, New York. She had only a few months of schooling during the summers as a child, and no formal art training at all. At age 12 she left her parents' farm and was hired as a servant. She married Thomas Moses in 1887 and worked with him in farming, first in the Shenandoah Valley of Virginia and later in upstate New York. Like many women of her time, she was frequently pregnant, giving birth to ten children, five of whom died in infancy.

Anna Moses began cultivating her artistic side after her husband's death in 1927, when she began serious embroidery. But arthritis forced her to abandon sewing, and she switched to painting. By sheer luck, several of her paintings were on display in a drugstore window in Hoosick Falls, New York, in 1931, where an art collector driving through the area chanced upon them. He bought up all the extant Moses paintings. Her appeal—she was 80, she was self-taught, and her work was very accessible to the general public—led to an exhibition at the Museum of Modern Art in New York City in 1939. By the time of her death at age 100, Anna "Grandma" Moses had produced about two thousand paintings. She continues to be a pillar of Americana, a genuine "folk" artist in the mold of Norman Rockwell.[6]

For the majority of older people, whether they continue their life's work, start a new career, or seek entirely new activities, the key to finding meaning in old age is involvement with community. The MacArthur Foundation Study of Successful Aging found that 80 percent of older Americans agreed that "life is not worth living if one cannot contribute to the well-being of others." Fully 60 percent of those interviewed for a study on "the new face of retirement" said that "feeling valued and needed" is extremely important to them.[7] These views corroborate Erik Erikson's theory of the stages of development, in which old age is a period of "generativity." Successful old age demands that looking outside oneself and concerns for the next generation triumph over stagnation and self-absorption.[8] But there simply aren't enough opportunities in contemporary America for the kind of productive engagement that my mother cherishes and that the Landaus, Daniel Schorr, and Grandma Moses all represent. Vigorous older people need challenging employment or stimulating volunteer positions or important caregiving responsibilities. They don't want to "disengage" from society; rather, they want to use their experience, their knowledge, and their wisdom to make contributions they couldn't have made earlier in life.

Very gradually, programs are developing that recognize these needs of the elderly, as well as the complementary needs of the most vulnerable members of society. Civic Ventures, a non-profit organization dedicated to creating outlets for older people, sees the elderly as a major untapped resource for a society desperately in need of greater civic engagement. One of its projects is Foster Grandparents, which pairs an older person with an inner-city child. The program had a rocky start. First proposed in the 1960s as a way for low-income older people to give one-on-one attention to needy children, it initially met with resistance from the agencies for the children themselves. They came up with an astonishing series of ever more ludicrous objections: The older adults might bring "diseases" to the children. Worse, they might molest the kids.[9] Ultimately, sanity prevailed, and the program was established as a means to engage low-income older adults to work for minimum wage at least twenty hours per week. Today the program involves some 25,000 older Americans who interact with approximately 100,000 children each year. They work with teenage mothers, with abused children, with kids who are terminally ill. They offer advice, support, and companionship. Numerous studies of the outcomes of the program show that both the old and the young benefit from the interactions.

Another Civic Ventures program is the Experience Corps. Intended as a sort of domestic, geriatric version of the Peace Corps, it also had a slow start. Despite a six-month planning period, a distinguished advisory board, and the active involvement of physician-researchers such as the gerontologist Linda Fried from Johns Hopkins, recruitment for the program was painfully difficult.[10] What this program has done is to send retirees into inner-city elementary schools to serve as tutors and mentors to children. The initial pilot project created teams of fifteen half-time Experience Corps members who went into schools in five cities. In addition to tutoring one-on-one, they provided an extra set of hands so that the regular teachers could give their students individualized attention. The older volunteers proved to be reliable and dedicated. Both the children and their tutors benefited: one study found that 68 percent of the men and women who participated said they had learned new skills, and 74 percent said they had grown personally.[11] They reported that working on a regular basis gave structure to their lives, afforded them a sense of purpose, and provided them with a new extended social network made up of the other Corps members. Today there are 1,300 Experience Corps participants in twelve cities, working with thousands of children in this small but dynamic experiment in intergenerational renewal.[12]

Robust elders are limited in their quest for a meaningful old age by the paucity of positions—there just aren't very many options for productive engagement. But for frail elders, the prospects for finding meaning in their lives are even more limited. Over and beyond worrying about the existence of suitable activities, they need to be concerned about flexibility in their work: they may have limited endurance and couldn't work for eight hours straight, maybe not even for four hours. They need to be able to reach libraries or community centers or preschools—no mean feat if you have severe arthritis or impaired vision or advanced Parkinson's disease, particularly in suburbia, where it's hard to go anywhere without a car. They can't simply drive off to the local elementary school to tutor in the after-school program. They can't hope to start a new career in carpentry. Frail elders often view the retirement years as an endless series of medical appointments, punctuated by a rare visit with children and grandchildren. They are socially isolated, they feel superannuated and, not surprisingly, they frequently suffer from depression. If octogenarians are going to be able to find meaning in old age, along with the "young old," we will need to develop a more reciprocal, interdependent, and communitarian world view.

ON THE basis of what I had read about Wanda Ford in her medical record, I expected to find a wreck. I could visualize her before I entered the room at the skilled nursing facility, or transitional care unit, where she was recuperating after a week-long hospital stay. She had gone to the local emergency room because she couldn't breathe and was having palpitations. She had been found to have a flare-up of her chronic congestive heart failure, which caused fluid to build up in her lungs. Wanda also had had a rapid, irregular heartbeat, necessitating multiple strong medications to control it. The fact that she had a kind of cancer—multiple myeloma—and tended to be anemic didn't help matters. She needed every molecule of oxygen she could get, but she was running low on red blood cells, the transport vehicles for oxygen, which compounded the burden on her already weakened heart.

As soon as the doctors had gotten most of the excess fluid out of Wanda's system, slowed her heart with a combination of medications, and transfused her with a couple of pints of blood, they had discharged her to the skilled facility where I worked. I expected she would be wearing oxygen, piped in from the wall through plastic tubing and into prongs inserted in her nostrils. She would most likely still have an intravenous catheter in her arm, since she had been getting supplementary doses of potent diuretics whenever the fluid began accumulating in her lungs or her legs. I imagined she would have multiple bruises on her arms, the nearly universal mark of a hospital admission. She would be wearing a blue-and-white johnny, standard institutional garb. And she would be lying in bed, propped up on three pillows, the only way she could breathe easily. She might still have a catheter in her bladder so the nurses could accurately measure her urine output.

When I knocked on Wanda's door and entered her sunny room in the nursing home, I wasn't sure which of the four women in loose-fitting slacks and flowery blouses was the patient. None of them appeared sick and no one looked like 75, the age listed in Wanda's chart. The woman sitting on the edge of the bed seemed like the most plausible candidate for patienthood, despite the prayer book on her lap and the exuberant chatter streaming from her mouth. "Mrs. Ford?" I asked tentatively.

"That's me," the woman on the bed acknowledged, turning toward me.

"I'm Dr. Gillick," I introduced myself. "I wasn't expecting a crowd." She laughed, a great big belly laugh, and told me her visitors were her "church sisters." I indicated that I needed to spend a few minutes with Mrs. Ford to speak with her and examine her as part of the routine admissions process of the transitional care unit. The three other women nodded at me, evidently giving me permission to go about my business, but showed no signs of leaving. They smiled and resumed their conversation, focusing on each other rather than on Wanda.

Despite her robust appearance, Wanda Ford was a very sick woman. She had cardiomyopathy, a progressive weakening of the heart muscle, which led to both mechanical and electrical problems. Her heart did not pump well, which caused fluid to back up in unfortunate places, and the electrical currents did not flow properly, resulting in an irregular heart rhythm. Her recent hospitalization had been her third this year, and it was only June. She was not one to neglect her health: she took all her medications as prescribed, though her regimen was so complicated that she had to consult a neatly printed set of directions to figure out what pills to take. Each time she visited her primary care physician, which she did every few weeks, and each time she was hospitalized, the doctors changed one or two of her medications.

Getting to and from all her medical appointments was not easy. She got winded too quickly to manage public transportation; she found "The Ride," a service provided by the local Elder Services Agency, to be unreliable; and taxis were prohibitively expensive. But Wanda had a great many friends, and some of them drove. For a while, when she had been getting daily radiation therapy treatments for the painful lesions in her bones, an old friend from her days selling subway tokens drove her to the hospital and waited for her while she underwent the 15-minute treatment.

Buying groceries was also a challenge. Wanda lived on the first floor of a triple-decker together with her 40-year-old son, who had Down syndrome. He helped around the house, vacuuming and doing the dishes, but he was not able to make change or read a shopping list. Wanda relied on her upstairs neighbor, who assured her that picking up a few extra items when she bought groceries for herself and her four children was no trouble. And then there were the church sisters.

Wanda didn't think she could survive without the church. In addition to providing concrete help, such as doing her laundry and picking up her ever-changing prescriptions from the drugstore, the sisters prayed with her, sang hymns with her, and literally held her hand through all her trials. It wasn't a one-way street: Wanda herself, she confessed shyly, was a "missionary" for the church. She explained that meant that she visited the sick and tried to give them courage and hope. She told the old people—at 75, she didn't think of herself as in the same camp—that they had nothing to fear because the Lord was watching over them.

"Something you have to remind yourself of, too," I commented during a subsequent visit when Wanda was discouraged by her slow progress.

She smiled. "I know. But He is looking after me, too."

"Except maybe when he's on vacation," I replied.

"Oh no," Wanda responded, becoming more animated. "He doesn't take vacations."

"Maybe a little nap now and then," I suggested.

Wanda laughed. "I have wondered about that sometimes," she admitted.

Although she had lightened up a bit, Wanda still seemed sad. I assumed she was dismayed because her breathing remained labored and her ankles were still swollen despite a week in the hospital and a week in the skilled nursing facility. But she was worried about her son: "I was hoping to be home by now. I don't like to leave my son by himself for so long."

Joseph was 40. All the neighbors knew him, and church members checked to make sure he was all right. "He's a good boy," his mother told me, "but he's simple. You know, simple in the head. He was born that way. I was 34 when I became pregnant with him. They told me his type of problem was common with older women, women over 35. But I guess my eggs were old at 34. Now, I'm afraid people will take advantage of him. He's so good-natured. He'll do whatever you tell him to. I used to give him money every week until I discovered he was giving it all to homeless alcoholics. They learned I gave him something after I cashed my paycheck each week, so a different man would come to him after every payday. They didn't threaten him or hold him up—they just asked real nicely, and he gave all his money away. Since then I try to make sure he doesn't carry more than a couple of dollars around. He's an easy mark."

We talked a little more. I asked whether Wanda had chosen a health care proxy, since evidently her son was not able to fulfill that role. She had. I asked whether she would want attempted cardiopulmonary resuscitation if her heart stopped. She said she would. But suddenly she told me that she was ready to go to Heaven whenever the Lord called her. She wasn't afraid. She was looking forward to being someplace where life was easier, where she could always catch her breath. And, she commented wryly, she would be glad not to have so many doctors' appointments. Her one worry was her son: he was the main reason she clung to life "on this side," as she put it.

Joseph, as it turned out, was not merely a source of worry for his mother. He was the joy of her life. A single mother, she had raised him alone. She had worked as a token collector, then as a supervisor for the transit authority. She had also managed to serve as Joseph's advocate, fighting for him to have suitable schooling in the time before Congress passed the Education of the Handicapped Act and long before the Americans with Disabilities Act.[13] Wanda had practically invented the term "special education" at the urban schools her son attended. She had been fearless, persistent, and ultimately, persuasive.

"Joseph is what makes all my aches and pains go away. I forget about my breathing." I may have looked skeptical, so she added, "For a little while, anyway. And looking out for him is something I can still do at 75. To run after a small child, a toddler, you have to be young yourself. For other kinds of work, like farming, you have to be physically strong. My parents grew up on a farm and started out as farmers until they moved up North. You can't do that kind of back-breaking labor if you have cardiomyopathy." That got my attention; I hadn't been sure just how much she knew or wished to know about her illness. "But you can do things for other people. We're all God's children. He's a loving Father, but—" she seemed stuck, not certain her logic was taking her where she wanted to go.

"But he delegates a lot of the hard work to his representatives on earth," I offered. Wanda nodded. That's what she was: God's representative on earth, working in her church and in her own family to make the world a better place.

WANDA FORD regarded old age as a time to devote to prayer and what she called missionary work, which was what other people just called visiting the sick. For the first time in decades, she had the time and the motivation to attend to her spiritual life. She viewed old age as a time to come to terms with her neighbors and with her God. She cherished the time she spent with her son, who as an adult with Down syndrome benefited enormously from her nurturing. She was fortunate to be a part of a faith-based community in her own neighborhood. Her church was within walking distance, as were most of the other church members she visited. And if her congestive heart failure got in the way of her walking even that short distance, other congregants would come to her or would drive her.

Membership in a faith community is one way of staying connected with other people. For many older individuals, it's not an option they would choose. But neither is the isolation of suburbia or the anonymity of city life. What's needed is a different kind of living arrangement altogether. A couple of radical architects came up with the idea of the planned community. Their idea was to deliberately design a whole town, using architecture to facilitate a sense of community. The visionary husband/wife architect team of Andres Duaney and Elizabeth Platter-Zyberk succeeded in implementing their ideas with the community of Seaside, Florida, a town they began developing in the early 1980s. Touted in the *Atlantic Monthly* as the answer to America's social problems, it embodies the principles of an alternative to suburban living. The town has a central green where key community institutions are housed; all the dwellings are within a five-minute walk of the town center; and a variety of stores are conveniently located along the town periphery. These principles became the core idea of what was labeled the "new urbanism." The aim was to create a "pedestrian village" built around a social space where people can gather, make friends, and talk.[14] Designed to combat suburban sprawl and to promote social interaction, such communities potentially enable older people to overcome isolation and anomie.

"New urban" developments might be good for all of us, but they are likely to be particularly good for older people. They solve the problems of inadequate transportation, and they foster social networks. But wholesale replacement of the American suburbs with new villages is not going to happen anytime soon, certainly not soon enough to give the baby boomers the environment we will need in order to thrive as we age. Another approach to fostering community, the intergenerational campus, seems a little more promising.

The idea of the intergenerational college campus stemmed as much from fiscal prudence as from idealism. It was born from the recognition that many universities have extraordinary but underutilized resources and need additional sources of revenue to survive. The typical college is only in session half the year (parents who shell out $40,000 a year or more for tuition, room, and board at private universities are painfully aware that their children are actually in school for a mere 28 or 30 weeks a year) and may not even have a summer session. Some colleges have found they can rent their facilities to summer camps or other special programs. A handful have chosen to build continuing-care retirement communities on site, enabling the elderly residents to take college courses alongside the adolescent population. The speakers who come to the campus, the concerts and movies that are offered, are open to both young and old. The hope is that the older people will serve as a resource for the students, providing the kind of information about careers that is lacking from the typical career counseling office. They can also act as surrogate grandparents, giving advice and encouragement that teenagers might reject if it came from their own parents.

The University of North Carolina at Asheville, for example, set up the Center for Creative Retirement. Founded in 1988, the Center doesn't actually provide housing on campus, but it puts together an extensive program for seniors to promote learning and volunteering. Its "College for Seniors" is separate from the regular classes offered to undergraduates. Instead, the Center's model is to draw on its own members' experience and professional expertise—with some involvement of university faculty—to teach courses to other older people. The students in the College for Seniors can take advantage of the university's facilities, such as the library and the gym. In the fall of 2004, the course offerings included "Gandhi in South Africa," "Concepts of Ecology," and "What Mortality Teaches" as well as "Growing Herbs" and "Tai Chi."[15]

The Center for Creative Retirement also coordinates an impressive series of community service programs. Working though the university's Career Center, it trains older people to serve as advisers to undergraduates who are looking for internship positions or trying to get a job or struggling to figure out what to do with themselves when they grow up. It also uses older volunteers to help staff an after-school computer lab for middle school students, and members of the Center help organize regional science competitions.

A small college outside Boston has taken a different approach. Lasell College chose to build a continuing-care retirement community on its campus. Structured like a New England town, with a town hall at its center, Lasell Village has fourteen interconnected buildings that house 210 independent older people. The community has its own skilled nursing facility on site in case its residents need short-term, intensive rehabilitation or medical care. Lasell's approach to "lifelong learning" is to require its residents to commit to and complete (if they can) 450 hours of an individualized educational program each year. The institution is serious about its mission: it has hired a full-time academic dean to help students choose how to fulfill the educational requirements. They can do this in a variety of ways, ranging from enrolling in a course at Lasell to attending special courses for the Village residents to mentoring Lasell College students. Traveling and studying in an Elderhostel program counts toward the requirement, as does volunteering in the college's day care center. A non-profit organization, Lasell Village has also established the Fuss Center for Research on Aging and Intergenerational Studies to evaluate its own and other approaches to aging.

Settings like those I've just described—a faith community, a planned community, or an intergenerational campus community—promote the development of relationships and facilitate finding meaningful work. They all involve creating social capital, the social networks that are so sorely lacking in much of American society.[16] But for the frail elderly, even these environments may not be enough. To make sure that a good old age remains an option even into the eighties and nineties, we will need to utilize technology. With computers, for instance, we can create virtual communities. For older people with mobility problems or with medical conditions that limit their attention span, the Internet offers several intriguing possibilities for establishing new kinds of reciprocal relationships.

The Web can enable older people to be in contact with many other adults whom they will never see or speak to. Just as many vigorous older people have successfully mentored in face-to-face situations, frail elders can learn to mentor online. And the mentoring doesn't have to be restricted to tutoring students. Several studies suggest that adults in the early stage of their careers benefit enormously from mentoring.[17] Typically their department chair (in academia) or their boss (in business) is far more interested in his own advancement than in that of his underlings. Not uncommonly, he uses the junior members of his staff, whether in a research lab or a law firm, to further his own projects. Occasionally, the interests of both are truly allied. But only rarely does the chief see his role as helping his staff develop their own areas of interest and expertise. Calling on retired professionals to mentor men and women early in their careers could partially compensate for the inadequacies of the existing system. And the beauty of Internet matchmaking is that it does not require geographic proximity.

Regardless of their physical limitations, older people will be able to market their services on the Internet. Right now the Internet is used principally to buy and sell material things, bringing together people who have something to sell with those who want to buy, whatever their location may be. Instead of the tedium of reading through want ads, squinting to make out the small print, struggling to decode the abbreviations, and being forced to move from one inky newspaper to another, we can simply enter key words. We can search at whatever time of day is convenient; we can often see a photograph of the object of interest; and we can make a deal instantly. The idea of selling services in a similar way is just starting to catch on. "Craigslist" now posts jobs in various cities from Boston to San Francisco, allowing for a similar match-making between buyer and seller without the intermediary of an employment agency or a human resources department. With a little ingenuity, an Internet entrepreneur could capitalize on the untapped potential of tens of thousands of older people with services to offer. Advice is the obvious service, but older people could also proofread term papers or provide feedback on college assignments or even facilitate Internet support groups.

Although the current crop of octogenarians use e-mail to communicate with their children and grandchildren, most of them did not enter old age with sophisticated computer skills. By 2025, however, seniors will be equipped with far more word-processing and spreadsheet expertise. They will be able to surf the Web long after they've had to give up surfing the ocean. They will be able to format newsletters and maintain databases and undertake searches even if they have trouble hearing and difficulty walking. They will be able to use their expertise both to remain independent, ordering groceries and pharmaceuticals online, for instance, and also to remain active participants in their communities.

IN ORDER to have a good old age, we will need to remain productive members of society. We will need work, not just play. And we will need not only to find suitable work, but also to be able to get to places of work or bring them to us. Society will have to be restructured—physically and psychologically—to allow for flexible hours and to accommodate people with impaired hearing, poor vision, and limited mobility. The major obstacle to making this possible is not inadequate infrastructure, although that is a problem, nor the absence of political will, though that's another problem. The true barrier is our deep-seated faith in individualism.

Americans tend to define success, happiness, and well-being in terms of personal fulfillment. We have built our towns assuming the primacy of the individual over the community. And as a corollary to our belief in individualism, we hold autonomy, or control over our lives, to be sacrosanct: "Freedom, liberty, autonomy, choice, personal rights, voluntarism, and finally empowerment are now the most often used and revered words in our moral and civil discourse."[18] This trend toward enshrining autonomy—literally "self-rule"—dates to the late 1970s. In his survey of American values, Daniel Yankelovich found that America in the 1970s was moving from a culture of self-denial to one of self-fulfillment, just as the first baby boomers reached their mid- to late thirties. A recent study of the American middle class by Alan Wolfe suggests that the baby boomers are becoming increasingly preoccupied with their own affairs. And Robert Putnam, in his seminal work

Bowling Alone, identifies autonomy as the sacred cow of the generation born after World War II, in contrast to the civic-mindedness of the "greatest generation."[19]

Belief in the preeminence of autonomy creates problems for all strata of society. Willard Gaylin and Bruce Jennings have suggested that "autonomy now preempts civility, altruism, paternalism, beneficence, community, mutual aid, and other civil values that essentially tell a person to set aside his own interests in favor of the interests of other people or the good of something larger than himself." These other principles have a place in building a moral civilization: "Our humanity is fulfilled by conjoining rights and responsibilities, autonomy and relationships, independence and interdependence."[20] This culture of autonomy is not only problematic for society as a whole, but it fails abysmally in meeting the needs of old age. Older people may have to rely on others for help with the most mundane activities, such as dressing or showering. They may no longer have the intellectual capacity, the physical strength, or the endurance to carry on with their earlier work. They may not have the energy, the ambition, or the wherewithal to embark on a new career. To have a good old age, we are going to have to think of ourselves less as isolated atoms and more as molecules—parts of compounds that combine with other compounds to produce new and marvelous substances.

Excessive emphasis on autonomy has brought us a slew of problems. Not only is it an impediment to the creation of meaningful work for older people, but it is also the source of widespread use of near-futile medical treatments toward the end of life and underlies the small but growing interest in physician-assisted suicide. Sadie Solomon's daughters (Chapter 3) insisted that their 90-year-old mother go to the hospital, where she was attached to a respirator, transfused with blood, and flooded with fluids before she died. They were asked about how to proceed because physicians have turned every medical intervention into a potential choice, even when there is no meaningful choice to be made. In their rejection of the medical paternalism of the 1950s, responding to the rightful recognition that many decisions about treatment are value-laden and not merely technical, doctors have ended up leaving patients with too much choice. They have placed burdens on families that they do not want to bear instead of owning up to their own responsibility to guide care, all in the name of autonomy.[21] As Franz Ingelfinger, a gastroenterologist and former editor of the *New England Journal of Medicine,* put it when he developed esophageal cancer and was given nothing but a litany of options by his doctors:

> The physician should recommend a specific course of action. He must take the responsibility, not shift it onto the shoulders of the patient. The patient may then refuse the recommendation, which is perfectly acceptable, but the physician who would not use his training and experience to recommend the specific action to a patient . . . does not warrant the somewhat tarnished but still distinguished title of doctor.[22]

An excessive belief in the value of autonomy has also contributed to the interest in physician-assisted suicide. Death is the final threat to autonomy—it's bad enough that after we die, we will no longer have control over anything, but it's unthinkable that we should have no control over when and how we die. When Jay Robinson's daughters came to me with a plea to help end their father's suffering (Chapter 3), they were desperately afraid of losing control and thought that physician-assisted suicide was the way to hold onto it. They saw physician-assisted suicide as a means for their father to decide when to end his life, aided and abetted by a physician who would give him the pharmacological means to achieve his end. The notion that there are certain things over which none of us has control—such as what we die of and when we go—was foreign to them. What they came to understand was that their father could die well, that he could die with a modicum of dignity and without pain, even without exercising absolute control over his death. He could influence small things, such as the dose of his medications and whether he was at home or in a residential hospice or in a hospital at the end, and those small decisions would have to suffice.

Excessive adherence to autonomy encourages the baby boomers to demand painful and useless treatments; it prompts some to resort to suicide when those treatments fail; and it teaches us that we should seek personal fulfillment even in our final days. Only a radical change in attitude will allow tomorrow's octogenarians to accept limits on medical treatment, to endorse palliative care at the end of life, and to enjoy their final years in an environment that is truly conducive to fulfillment.

Finale

THE BABY BOOMER generation has a choice to make. We can stumble into old age, hoping that our physicians will have the wisdom to treat us appropriately, given our degree of vigor or of infirmity, and expecting to accept their beneficence. We can go about our business today, assuming that our politicians, guided by health policy mavens, will see fit to truly overhaul Medicare so that it provides coordinated care combined with compassion and continuity. And we can blithely assume that housing options will evolve spontaneously, guaranteeing us attractive apartments with every possible high-tech convenience, in an ultra-modern assisted living facility or nursing home, should we need to move to such a place. In short, we can remain optimistic because we believe that abiding by the latest dietary recommendations and adhering to a regular exercise regimen will suffice to keep us healthy and strong until, at age 100, we die in our sleep.

Alternatively, the baby boomers can decide individually and collectively to do our utmost to shape our future. Since passivity has not been a characteristic widely attributed to the generation born between 1946 and 1964, it is surprising that acquiescence is precisely what we've seen to date. Perhaps our reticence arises from our terror at the prospect of death, which is after all the culmination of aging. But while death has poked its head out of the closet, with the rousing success of books such as Sherwin Nuland's *How We Die*, aging has stayed safely tucked away on the top shelf, dusty and out of view. Maybe the acknowledgment that before death comes a no-man's-land in which many people merely exist—unproductive, unvalued, and often unwell, but alive—is just too mind-boggling to consider. We need to act to landscape that terrain so that it is not barren and desolate, but rather a period of fulfilled yearning, triumphant aspiration, but also sadness and grief—much like all the other phases of life.

What exactly am I urging my fellow boomers to do? What I am suggesting is that we need to change our attitudes, our behavior, and many of our social institutions. Some of the actions we should take can occur in the privacy of a voting booth or in a physician's office. We can vote for candidates for political office who support substantive Medicare reform—though we may need to run for office ourselves to find such a candidate. We can ask to be involved in the management of our chronic illnesses and to be tested for common conditions like hearing impairment when we go to the doctor. Other actions will require a more coordinated and concerted effort. We need to persuade our communities to build housing for older people that is guided by a philosophy of respectful, person-centered care; we should push businesses and academia to develop meaningful positions for older individuals;

and we need to reward philanthropic organizations that support innovative projects designed to integrate older people into the wider society.

For starters, we need to recognize that as a group, we have extraordinary power. There are 77 million Americans who were born between 1946 and 1964. As of the year 2000, we accounted for 27.5 percent of the population. Our annual spending power is estimated at $2.2 trillion, equally divided between the nearly 24 million households headed by younger boomers, those born between 1956 and 1964, and older boomers, born between 1946 and 1955, who account for the remaining 22 million households. We have achieved higher levels of education than any previous generation. Not only do we spend money, not only are we educated, but we also vote. In the 2000 presidential election, 59 percent of the eligible electorate voted, but 69 percent of older boomers cast ballots.[1] Our voices matter, although we may need to speak in unison to be heard.

Once we stop burying our heads in the sand, we should make a few crucial changes in personal behavior. In particular, we will need to get moving and exercise. Physical activity is one way that individuals can make a difference in their own health. Exercise has three main salutary effects. First, it markedly decreases the risk of heart disease, its best-known benefit. Heart disease continues to be the leading cause of death in people over age 65 despite cardiopulmonary resuscitation, coronary care units, stents, and cholesterol-lowering medications. Regular exercise can also help prevent obesity, which is increasingly recognized as an epidemic in twenty-first-century America. People who exercise regularly are rarely overweight, and people who are overweight can only hope to lose weight if they eat less and exercise more. None of the fad diets that have gripped our imagination over the last decade have been able to surmount the basic laws of thermodynamics. Finally—and this is probably the least-recognized positive consequence of exercise—older people who remain fit tend to stay self-sufficient.[2] That means that they can dress themselves, go to the bathroom on their own, and bathe without help, and they are self-reliant in areas such as cooking, cleaning, and shopping. In short, walking briskly for half an hour three to five times a week can help stave off a variety of infirmities that make it hard for older people to engage in the aspects of life that they find most meaningful.

We should keep moving, but we probably should not make quite so many geographic moves. When we constantly resettle in new locations, thinking nothing of spending a few years in Chicago and then a few more in Seattle and next in Chapel Hill, we never establish roots. Cultivating relationships with family and friends not only mitigates against loneliness, but also has an effect on health. Patients who, despite their best efforts at eating right and exercising, suffer a stroke or heart attack recover more quickly and are more likely to survive the acute episode altogether if they have frequent social contacts. The same is true after a hip fracture. And while dementia, the great plague of old age, is principally due to abnormal brain chemistry, social engagement does seem to help in delaying its onset and minimizing its impact.[3]

It is not only our behavior that needs to be modified, but also our attitudes. For years we have had drilled into us the virtue of screening tests—blood cholesterol levels, mammograms, prostate specific antigen tests. Not all Americans follow the recommended screening guidelines, nor do their physicians. But those who do will need to change their stance as they age and develop life-limiting diseases. We will need to stop obsessing about things that no longer matter, resisting the impulse to request Pap smears and PSA tests, and start paying attention to new areas that do matter. Falling and breaking a hip presents a far greater threat to independence and happiness at age 85 than does cervical cancer.

We are also going to have to change our attitude toward medical care. We need to abandon the view that medicine is either relentlessly curative or exclusively palliative; instead, it can lie between these two extremes, focusing on quality of life. A desire for treatment that allows us to see and hear and to think and walk is perfectly compatible with an interest in treatment that prolongs life—sometimes. We have to accept the painful need to make trade-offs, recognizing that some kinds of potentially life-extending therapy are incompatible with remaining independent, lucid, and comfortable.

Finally—and this is the most difficult attitudinal change— baby boomers will need to give up our single-minded devotion to individual autonomy and to accept the fact that community is tremendously important as we age. Older people increasingly define themselves in terms of their relationships to family and friends and to the surrounding society. The elderly also depend on family, friends, and others in their community to facilitate the exercise of their autonomy: if they are to continue to be able to make choices about their lives, they need others to help them implement their decisions.[4]

All these changes in attitudes and behavior will not come easily, so we will need to develop ways to facilitate them. It is unrealistic and unreasonable to expect that individuals should simply take greater responsibility for their own health, for example, without giving them the tools for doing so. Even though science is one of the fastest-developing fields today, there is no systematic effort to educate adults about science and medicine once they leave high school or college. During the entire 65 years that the average high school graduate has remaining to him, he is left to rely on the media and his physician for up-to-date, unbiased, comprehensive health information. The professions—whether nursing, teaching, or law—require continuing education credits to retain certification; but in the domain of everyday health, no ongoing formal instruction is either expected or available. To compensate for this glaring deficiency, the medical profession could offer weeklong seminars (conceivably at resorts, featuring a mixture of work and play), or ongoing series of evening lectures, or online educational programs on topics such as cancer screening, the perils of hypertension, and devising an exercise regimen. These courses would not be compulsory, nor would failure to participate be punishable by a fine (analogous to failure to wear a seatbelt in some states), but Medicare or senior health maintenance organizations could offer a premium rebate for annual attendance.

One could argue that we should have access to formal instruction about other aspects of life as well—economics, politics, and the law, for example. But health is a special case because the information is complex and rapidly evolving, and the consequences of ignorance are potentially devastating.[5] And while existing state-run educational programs, such as driver's education and anti-drug seminars, are notoriously tedious and have not been shown to be effective, what I am proposing is a multitude of programs, designed by physicians and certified by Medicare. In this instance, market forces could potentially stimulate the development of high-quality "products," with enough diversity to appeal to a variety of consumers.

In a similar vein, if exercise is important, we should create incentives to encourage it. Exercise has the tremendous advantage that, unlike prescription drugs, it is cheap, but the disadvantage that, again unlike medication, it is difficult to take. Swallowing a pill is considerably easier than traveling to the local health club to work out, or swimming at the community pool, or even peddling on a stationary bicycle in one's own home. Putting exercise equipment in senior centers along with providing free transportation to the center would facilitate exercise. An even more potent stimulus would be a system of accumulating points ("Prolific Peddling Points"), analogous to Frequent Flier miles, which could be credited toward the price of prescription drugs or the cost of subscribing to part B of Medicare (coverage for physician services and laboratory tests) or could result in a discount on a MediGap policy. Medicare would in effect subsidize the costs for enrollees who engaged in effective health promotion. Each Medicare recipient would receive a password that would enable him to "sign in" whenever he used an exercise bicycle equipped with a special meter to record his performance. Approved "weigh-in" centers might allow seniors to assess whether they were within a narrow range of their predetermined target weight, with additional "points" awarded annually (or more often) for achieving the desired weight.

In addition to personal changes, we will also need to develop new institutions, in the broadest sense. In particular, we will have to create better residential environments for older people with disabilities. Nursing homes and assisted living facilities should be conceived of as variants of a single, resident-centered model. This model will seek to promote the highest quality of life for its residents, not just to maximize their physical safety, which is what so much of nursing care is about today. To that end, we will have to create places to live that are true communities—where the residents feel that they are part of a larger society and that they have work to do, a contribution to make, as well as the opportunity to enjoy themselves. Jobs in those communities will have to be flexible to accommodate the needs of both older workers and their caregivers.

If we hope to have people available to take care of us as we age, we're going to have to redefine caregiving jobs to make them attractive. That will mean boosting pay, increasing the prestige associated with such jobs, and creating avenues for advancement. Since we still won't have enough people to provide hands-on care for all the older people who will need help in areas like dressing and bathing, we will have to come to the assistance of family caregivers. Family members already provide the bulk of this kind of care, but they will need more flexibility on the job if they are to do more, given that they already have other jobs as well as their own families. In short, we will have to restructure the workplace.

If we want to keep older people out of nursing homes altogether, we need to find ways to emulate village life. The suburban model, in which people need to drive to reach stores, jobs, and civil institutions, is isolating for older people with disabilities, and rural existence is equally problematic. Cities are increasingly appealing to older individuals, but for those who can't stand the pace, noise, dirt, or crime of urban life, a community with a true intergenerational atmosphere, such as a retirement center integrated into a college campus, is a good alternative.

New institutions—whether they are nursing homes, communities, or places of work—need to be nurtured in order to grow. Just as incentives can stimulate attitudinal and behavioral changes, similarly, legislation and regulations can foster institutional development. We will need to enact comprehensive Medicare reform if our health care system is to be reshaped to promote chronic disease management rather than crisis care. Ideally, we would design several variants of Medicare to provide the optimum set of benefits for older people, recognizing that some elders are robust, some are frail, and some are dying, and that each group has vastly different needs. And we need to focus on quality-of-life issues: as long as the regulators scrutinize nursing homes for their attention to health and safety rather than to the quality of life of their residents, we will continue to have sterile pseudo-hospitals masquerading as "homes" for the elderly.

What will motivate us to engage in the political process to reform our institutions? It is crucial that we see examples of the possible all around us—pilot projects, demonstration projects, and above all stories, tales of the difference that better nursing homes and dynamic intergenerational campuses can make. Those stories will come from our parents and our neighbors; they will be told in books like this one. In order to have the widest possible effectiveness, these stories of life's potential, and the ways the environment can either trample or enhance that potential, will need to become the stuff of the media. We need an outpouring of news articles and human-interest stories in the press, on radio, and on television. And we will also need to see the dramas of old age played out on commercial television.

The pundits have long suspected that entertainment television is a major source of health information—or misinformation— for the general public. A study published in the *New England Journal of Medicine* in the mid-1990s looked at the portrayal of cardiopulmonary resuscitation on three leading TV medical dramas—*ER, Chicago Hope,* and *Rescue 911.* In the 97 episodes the authors watched, they observed 60 cases of attempted CPR, fully 75 percent of which were successful.[6] Patients literally got up off their stretchers, walked out of the emergency room, and went home. CPR was used primarily in the setting of trauma, and its principal beneficiaries were children, teenagers, and younger adults. In actuality, CPR is utilized most often in middle-aged or older people who have heart problems, and fewer than 10 percent survive. Among people over age 70 who sustain a cardiac arrest outside the hospital, fewer than 1 percent survive.[7]

Not only are television viewers presented with health information, but they are actually influenced by what they see. A fascinating survey of *ER* viewers found that over half reported learning about health issues from watching the show. Many of them said they discussed the issues raised on television with their friends, and a third of the respondents asserted that the health information they received helped them in their personal decision making. Nearly 15 percent claimed to have contacted a physician about a health problem because of what they saw on *ER*.[8]

Commercial television has the potential to capture much that is important in health policy debates. Yet another study that analyzed the health policy content of four shows during the 2000–2001 season *(ER, City of Angels, Gideon's Crossing,* and *Strong Medicine)* identified 127 "health policy interactions" in 74 episodes. Eleven percent of these dealt with end-of-life issues. Interestingly, among the issues that were *never* addressed were chronic illness, hospice care, nursing homes, and home care. Even in the realm of end-of-life issues, the programs dealt with refusal of treatment and with do-not-resuscitate orders, but not with quality-of-life concerns, advance directives, or physician-assisted suicide.[9]

News stories are another way to stimulate interest in the problems and challenges of old age. Public opinion polls indicate that people are very interested in health care policy stories, which should prompt further media attention. The amount of coverage devoted to health care policy issues is already increasing, though much of this attention remains focused on managed care. Health care costs in general and drug costs in particular, Medicare, and other economic issues remain the leading stories. While these articles help readers understand policy decisions, they rarely discuss the impact of policies on actual people. In one study, only a quarter of the articles on Medicare addressed the effect of legislation on individual patients or families.[10]

Even television advertisements can help bring the realities of aging to public consciousness. Right now, less than 3 percent of the fictional characters depicted on television, and an even smaller proportion of those featured in ads, are people over age 65. Women and minorities are particularly under-represented.[11] While a 30-second vignette intended to sell a product is hardly likely to capture the nuances of aging, the cumulative effect of increased attention to the facts about old age will help. As images of older people proliferate in the media—whether in medical dramas, health policy reports, or advertisements—we will begin to develop the kind of awareness of the issues necessary to bring about political change. And movie producers, novelists, memoirists, and artists are increasingly doing their share.[12]

The baby boomers have been reluctant to even think about our own old age, let alone to engage in the kinds of behavioral change and political activism I have discussed in this book. We don't want to think about aging because the prospect of losing bodily integrity, giving up our much-prized independence, and nearing the end of life's journey is terrifying to us. But perhaps we would not be so frightened if we developed a more balanced yet realistic view of what aging is or could be like. We tend to regard old age as hopelessly, irredeemably awful, and the only way we have come up with for dispelling this view is to try to transform it into its opposite—a period that is at once deeply fulfilling and endlessly entertaining. The truth is far more complex, textured, and fraught with possibility.

For nearly two hundred years, Americans have subscribed to this dualistic view of old age.[13] What has changed over time is the belief about just who is responsible for the horrors of old age and the related understanding of who has the power to mitigate them. In much of the nineteenth century, the individual was held responsible for his own decline. Gone was the ability to "hold opposites in creative tension, to accept the ambiguity, contingency, intractability, and unmanageability of human life" that had characterized early American culture. With the triumph of liberal individualism, self-control became a primary goal of existence. The maintenance of health and the accumulation of wealth were the markers of success. Victorian moralists disdained all those who in their old age were weak, poor, or dependent; in their view, "proper discipline" could enable individuals to remain healthy and self-reliant as they aged. But by the mid-twentieth century, the prevailing belief was that old age was inevitably marked by decay and dependence. The elderly were no longer blamed for their debility. They could, however, be rescued from ignominy through the beneficent intervention of social workers, physicians, and other gerontological technicians. Today, we have a new dualism in which old age is regarded as a period of disintegration, but one that can be delayed by means of dietary and exercise regimes, and that can be abolished entirely with genetic manipulation.

We need to see old age as neither all bad nor (when attacked with the appropriate weapons, whether by each of us individually or by trained professionals acting upon us collectively) all good, but rather, not unlike adolescence or other challenging stages of life, as both. Aging, Thomas Cole has said eloquently, "like illness and death, reveals the most fundamental conflict of the human condition: the tension between infinite ambition, dreams, and desires on the one hand, and vulnerable, limited, decaying physical existence on the other—the tragic and ineradicable conflict between body and spirit. This paradox cannot be eradicated by the wonders of modern medicine or by positive attitudes toward growing old."[14]

A solution to the dilemma of aging is to consider old age simultaneously as a time of meaning and spirituality, and as a time of sadness and loss. The purpose of this book is to portray the varieties of old age, with all their limitations as well as their possibilities. Its message is that we cannot overcome the inherent nature of old age, but we can transcend its infirmities through our attitudes, our behavior, and our institutions.

A good old age is within our grasp. Some have achieved it already, even without the benefit of the institutional changes that should, in the future, make it easier to attain. They have seized the opportunity to make something of their final years, usually through an intuitive understanding of the attitudinal and behavioral changes I have advocated. We know something about what works from a study carried out by the psychiatrist George Vaillant, who interviewed 800 older individuals to try to figure out what allowed them to find meaning and fulfillment as they aged. The most satisfied old people he interviewed cared about and reached out to other people, to whatever extent they could. They accepted their dependency, but maintained hope and believed in doing things for themselves if they could. They retained a sense of humor, took pleasure in their past achievements, and remained curious about the world. Most important, they retained contact and intimacy with old friends, continuously renewing their relationships: "And so in old age gardening becomes both a model and a metaphor for our waning lives. Good gardeners are by definition generative. With age they become . . . repositories of gardening lore. And in November they understand Integrity. They do not mourn the roses and tomatoes that are past. With satisfaction and good cheer they cover their dormant perennials with leaves, confident that in the future, they will rise again."[15]

Appendix

Notes

Acknowledgments

Index

Resources and References

THE MESSAGE of this book is that much has to change for the baby boomers to have a good old age. The necessary changes are within our grasp, but we will have to become better informed and to work with advocacy and reform organizations. Organizations and Web sites that offer information or seek to promote change are listed here, arranged according to the topic of each chapter. The descriptions of what the organizations do are taken directly from the Web sites listed.

PREVENTION

1. **The American Association of Retired Persons** is a non-profit, non-partisan membership organization of people over the age of 50 that is dedicated to enhancing quality of life with age. It seeks to help its members by providing information, advocacy, and service. It provides information about caregiving, health and

wellness, computers and technology, travel and leisure, as well as about public policy. In addition, AARP publishes a magazine *(AARP: The Magazine)* and a news bulletin *(AARP Bulletin)*, offers insurance, and has programs such as driver safety and tax assistance.

Web site: *www.aarp.org*
Address: 601 E. Street NW
Washington, DC 20049
Telephone: 1-888-687-2277

2. The Agency for Healthcare Research and Quality is a government agency that seeks to improve the quality, safety, efficiency, and effectiveness of health care for all Americans. Working under its direction is the U.S. Preventive Services Task Force, an independent panel of experts in primary care and prevention that systematically reviews evidence of effectiveness and develops recommendations for clinical preventive services (published as the "Guide to Clinical Preventive Services: A Report of the U.S. Preventive Services Task Force"). The AHRQ produces consumer versions of its practice guidelines, for example the "Pocket Guide to Staying Healthy at 50+", which can be downloaded from its Web site.

Web site: *www.ahrq.gov*
Address: John M. Eisenberg Building
540 Gaither Road
Rockville, MD 20850

3. The MIT AgeLab is based in MIT's School of Engineering. It draws on a multidisciplinary and global team of researchers, business partners, universities, and the aging community to design, develop, and deploy innovations to improve the quality of life. The Lab works in the areas of transportation, health, housing, communication, work and retirement, services, and decision making concerning aging and caregiving. It carries out projects on driving and personal mobility, wellness and self-empowered health, and independent living.

Web site: *http://web.mit.edu/agelab*
Address: 77 Massachusetts Avenue, Room E40-279
Cambridge, MA 02139
Telephone: 617-253-0253
E-mail: agelab-www@mit.edu

FRAILTY/CHRONIC DISEASE MANAGEMENT

1. The Program of All-Inclusive Care for the Elderly is a capitated managed care benefit for the frail elderly. It is intended for older individuals enrolled in both Medicare and Medicaid who are also eligible for admission to a nursing home. PACE uses a multidisciplinary team to provide and coordinate all needed preventive, primary, acute, and long-term-care services so that older individuals can continue living in the community. In addition to the PACE Web site, additional information is available through the government Web site, *www.cms.hhs.gov/pace.*

Web site: *www.npaonline.org*
Address: 801 North Fairfax Street, Suite 309
Alexandria, VA 22314
Telephone: 703-535-1565

2. Partnership for Solutions is an initiative led by the Johns Hopkins School of Public Health and the Robert Wood Johnson Foundation to improve the care and quality of life of people with chronic illness. It carries out research, communicates research findings to policymakers, business leaders, health professionals, and advocates, and works to identify promising solutions to problems faced by people with chronic illness. The project has developed programs to serve as models for people with chronic disease, including Faith in Action (a volunteer caregiver program) and Cash and Counseling (a demonstration project in three states that gives consumers flexibility in how they obtain care for chronic disease and supports informal caregivers).

Web site: *www.partnershipforsolutions.org*
Address: Johns Hopkins School of Hygiene and Public Health
Hampton House
624 North Broadway, Room 301
Baltimore, MD 21205
Telephone: 410-614-6059
E-mail: info@partnershipforsolutions.org

3. Family Caregiver Alliance offers information, education, services, research, and advocacy support to sustain families caring for people with chronic, disabling conditions. It publishes fact sheets on health conditions and legal issues, policy briefs, and a directory of caregiving programs. It established a National Center on Caregiving to advance the development of high-quality programs and policies for caregivers throughout the U.S.

Web site: *www.caregiver.org*
Address: 180 Montgomery Street, Suite 1100
San Francisco, CA 94104
Telephone: 415-434-3388
E-mail: info@caregiver.org

DEATH AND DYING

1. Growth House, Inc. seeks to improve the quality of compassionate care for people who are dying through public education and global professional collaboration. Its Web site includes sections on hospice care, palliative care, death with dignity, pain, and grief. It also provides disease-specific guides on caring for individuals with advanced heart failure, end-stage renal disease, and cancer.

Web site: *www.growthhouse.org*
Telephone: 415-863-3045
E-mail: info@growthhouse.org

2. The National Hospice and Palliative Care Organization is the largest non-profit membership organization representing hospice and palliative care programs and professionals in the United States. It is committed to improving end-of-life care and expanding access to hospice care with the goal of enhancing the quality of life for people dying in America and for their loved ones. The NHPCO has an ethics committee that addresses ethical issues in hospice and palliative care, a public policy committee to review and coordinate its lobbying work, and a standards committee to develop practice guidelines for hospices and palliative care programs. It puts out consumer brochures, including "Guide to Selecting a Hospice," "Guide to the Medicare Hospice Benefit," and "Guide to Communicating End-of-Life Wishes."

Web site: *www.nhpco.org*
Address: 1700 Diagonal Road, Suite 625
Alexandria, VA 22314
Telephone: 703-837-1500
E-mail: nhpco_info@nhpco.org

3. Americans for Better Care of the Dying (ABCD) is a non-profit organization that seeks to build momentum for reform, explore new methods and systems for delivering care, and shape public policy through evidence-based understanding. It reports news and events relating to end-of-life care and issues policy reports.

Web site: *www.abcd-caring.org*
Address: 3720 Upton Street, NW, Room B147
Washington, DC 20016
Telephone: 202-895-2660
E-mail: *info@abcd-caring.org*

MEDICARE

1. **Medicare—the Official U.S. Government Site for People with Medicare** provides information about all aspects of the Medicare program. Of particular use to consumers is the government handbook that details changes to Medicare and choosing a health plan: "Medicare and You 2006" (*www.medicare.gov/publication/ pubs/pdf/10050.pdf*). The entire Web site can be accessed in either English or Spanish.

Web site: *www.medicare.gov*
Telephone: 1-800-Medicare (1-800-633-4227)

2. **The Medicare Rights Center** is the largest independent source of Medicare information and assistance in the U.S. It helps older adults and people with disabilities find high-quality, affordable health care. The Center provides a telephone hotline service to answer questions about Medicare and has an education department to provide information about benefits and rights to people with Medicare as well as social workers, family members, and

health care providers. The Center is engaged in a public policy effort to bring the consumer voice to the national debate on Medicare reform.

Web site: *www.medicarerights.org*
Address: 1460 Broadway, 17th floor
New York, NY 10036
Telephone: 212-869-3850
E-mail: info@medicarerights.org

3. The Henry J. Kaiser Family Foundation is a non-profit, private foundation focusing on the major health care issues facing the United States. It is an independent voice and source of facts and analysis for policymakers, health care providers, and the general public. It develops and runs its own research and community programs, contracting with outside individuals and organizations to provide reliable information about the health care system. In particular, the Kaiser Foundation has put together a good overview, summary, and commentary about the Medicare Prescription Drug Improvement and Modernization Act of 2003, called "Talking About Medicare."

Web site: *www.kff.org*
Address: Kaiser Foundation Public Affairs Center
1330 G Street, NW
Washington, DC 20005
Telephone: 202-347-5270

Nursing Homes

1. The National Citizens' Coalition for Nursing Home Reform is made up of consumers and advocates who seek to achieve quality care for people with long-term care needs through informing and empowering consumers, by promoting best practices in care delivery, and by advocating for public policy responsive to consumer needs. It provides information and leadership on federal and state regulatory and legislative policy and promotes strategies to improve care for the residents of nursing homes.

Web site: *www.nccnhr.org*
Address: 1424 16th Street, NW, Suite 202
Washington, DC 20036
Telephone: 202-332-2275

2. Nursing Home Compare is a Web-based government service to help evaluate the quality of nursing homes. For each nursing home listed, it reports the number of nursing staff hours per resident per day and the number of deficiencies reported at the time of the most recent survey. It also provides information on quality indicators, which are meant to be used by consumers as potential warning signs of problems.

Web site: *www.medicare.gov/nhcompare*

3. The Pioneer Network is a not-for-profit organization that works to promote a new vision of nursing homes and a culture of aging that is life-affirming, humane, and meaningful. The network creates communication, networking, and learning opportunities. It identifies and promotes transformation in practices, service, public policy, and research. Pioneer offers publications, videos, a speakers bureau, an annual conference, and a newsletter, "Pioneer Networking," that describes its approach. It issued a guidebook in 2004, called "Getting Started: A Pioneering Approach to Culture Change in Long Term Care Organizations."

Web site: *www.pioneernetwork.net*
Address: P.O. Box 18648
Rochester, NY 14618
Telephone: 585-271-7570

4. The Eden Alternative brings together coalitions of people and organizations that are committed to creating better social and physical environments for people in nursing homes. It is dedicated to helping others create enlivening environments and to the elimination of the plagues of loneliness, helplessness, and boredom. This transformation occurs by seeing environments as habitats for human beings rather than as facilities for the frail and the elderly. The Eden Alternative sells audiotapes, videos, and booklets describing its approach, and publishes a newsletter.

Web site: *www.edenalt.com*
Address: 742 Turnpike Road
Sherburne, NY 13460
Telephone: 907-247-1197
E-mail: contact@edenalt.com

ASSISTED LIVING

1. The American Association of Homes and Services for the Aging (AAHSA) is committed to advancing the vision of healthy, affordable, and ethical aging services for Americans. It is intended for providers, professionals, businesses, and consumers. It advocates for public policy relating to long-term care and offers a list of publications and other resources.

Web site: *www.aahsa.org*
Address: 2519 Connecticut Avenue, NW
Washington, DC 20008
Telephone: 202-783-2242

2. The National Center for Assisted Living is the assisted living branch of the American Health Care Association, the nation's largest organization representing long-term care. It offers educational programs and public policy advocacy, lobbying at the state and federal levels. It has published "A Consumer's Guide to Assisted Living and Residential Care," as well as a monthly newsletter, "Focus," that covers business news, trends, regulatory activity, and legislative development, and provides examples of best practices in assisted living residences.

Web site: *www.ncal.org*
Address: 1201 L Street, NW
Washington, DC 20015
Telephone: 202-842-4444

Immortality/Longevity

1. **The New England Centenarian Study** grew out of the belief that centenarians are a select group of people who have a history of aging relatively slowly and who have either markedly delayed or entirely escaped diseases normally associated with aging, such as Alzheimer's disease, cancer, stroke, and heart disease. The NECS is principally engaged in conducting studies of longevity and the genetics of aging.

Web site: *www.bumc.bu.edu/centenarian*
Address: 715 Albany Street
Boston, MA 02118
Telephone: 617-638-6688

2. **The International Longevity Center–USA** is a not-for-profit, nonpartisan research, policy, and educational organization. Its mission is to help societies address the issues of population aging and longevity in positive and constructive ways. It has four distinct programs: research, communication, partnerships, and visiting scholars.

Web site: *www.ilcusa.org*
Address: 60 East 86th Street
New York, NY 10029
Telephone: 212-288-1468
E-mail: *info@ilcusa.org*

3. **The McGowan Institute for Regenerative Medicine** was established by the University of Pittsburgh School of Medicine and the Pittsburgh Medical Center to serve as a national center of expertise in regenerative medicine, focused on developing and delivering technologies that re-establish tissue and organ growth. The Institute seeks to generate scientific knowledge and to share that knowledge with researchers, clinicians, and the public through educational activities, training, and publications. It also supports commercialization of technologies to accelerate the translation of research discoveries into clinical treatment.

Web site: *www.mirm.pitt.edu*
Address: 100 Technology Drive, Suite 200
Pittsburgh, PA 15219
Telephone: 412-235-5100
E-mail: *McGowan@pitt.edu*

FINDING MEANING IN OLD AGE/RETIREMENT

1. **The Retirement Living Information Center** was established to assist seniors in living out their retirement years. It provides information about retirement communities and senior housing, new retirement communities as they arise, and state aging agencies. It maintains a list of great places to retire, including college towns and college-linked retirement communities.

Appendix

Web site: *www.retirementliving.com*
Address: 19 Ledgewood Road
Redding, CT 06896
Telephone: 203-938-0417
E-mail: *info@retirementliving.com*

2. Civic Ventures is a non-profit organization that seeks to expand the contribution of older Americans to society and to help transition the aging of America into a source of individual and social renewal. It is devoted to developing ways for older people to remain involved with their communities and to find meaning in life. It has sponsored the Experience Corps and Foster Grandparents, both of which enable older Americans to provide public service as tutors and mentors to children in urban settings.

Web site: *www.civicventures.org*
Address: 139 Townsend Street, Suite 505
San Francisco, CA 94107
Telephone: 415-430-0141
E-mail: *info@civicventures.org*

3. The Retirement Research Foundation is the nation's largest private foundation devoted solely to serving the needs of older Americans and enhancing their quality of life. It supports programs that improve services and care for the elderly, educate policymakers regarding the needs of elders, and expand employment and volunteer opportunities for older people. In particular, it has supported projects to enable older adults to live at home or in residential settings that facilitate independent living, and it has taken advantage of the wisdom and experience of older adults to promote community involvement.

Web site: *www.rrf.org*
Address: 8765 W. Higgins Road, Suite 430
Chicago, IL 60631
Telephone: 773-714-8080
E-mail: info@rrf.org

Notes

Prelude

1. This is not his real name. The patients described in this book are all composites, except for the members of my family. Each composite patient is based on a core patient for whom I have provided care, with features of other patients added both to protect the identity of the core patient and to allow me to make additional didactic points.

2. Caroline Fleck, "Pills, Potions, and Powders: Anti-Aging Compounds with Dubious Claims Proliferate," American Association of Retired Persons, November 2001, *www.aarp.org/bulletin/departments/2001;* Julia Sommerfield, "Time in a Bottle: Science or Scams?" MSNBC News, *www.msnbc.com.*

3. Among the most prominent titles are David Simon and Chopra Deepak, *Grow Younger, Live Longer: 10 Steps to Reverse Aging* (New York: Harmony Press, 2001), and Jean Carper, *Stop Aging Now! The Ultimate Plan for Staying Young and Reversing the Aging Process* (New York: Harper Perennial Library, 1996); see also Michael Brickey, *Defy Aging: Develop the Mental and Emotional Vitality to Live Longer, Healthier, and Happier Than You Ever Imagined* (New York: New Resources, 2000).

4. S. Jay Olshansky, Leonard Hayflick, and Bruce Carnes, "Position Statement on Human Aging," *Scientific American,* June 2002, *www.sciam .com.*

5. David Hackett Fischer, *Growing Old in America* (New York: Oxford University Press, 1978).

6. Betty Friedan, *The Fountain of Age* (New York: Simon and Schuster, 1993).

7. National Center for Health Statistics, *Health, United States, 1999: With Health and Aging Chartbook* (Hyattsville, Md., 1999).

8. For a discussion of the varieties of old age, see my book *Choosing Medical Care in Old Age: What Kind, How Much, When to Stop* (Cambridge, Mass.: Harvard University Press, 1994).

9. Thomas Cole, in his book *The Journey of Life: A Cultural History of Aging in America* (New York: Cambridge University Press, 1992), makes the point that America's "contemporary culture of aging is characterized . . . by the absence or inadequacy of shared meanings of old age" (p. xx). He stresses, too, that "scientific management" cannot solve the problem of old age. And Daniel Callahan, in his controversial book *Setting Limits* (New York: Simon and Schuster, 1987), makes a related point—that a good old age has more to do with meaning and less with longevity.

1. An Ounce of Prevention?

1. Luther Terry, the Surgeon-General responsible for the landmark report on smoking and health issued in 1964, began the transformative process. But it was Everett Koop whose flamboyance and cultivation of the media raised the office of the Surgeon-General to new heights. For the *Healthy People* report, see Centers for Disease Control and Prevention, National Center for Health Statistics, *Healthy People 2000* (Washington, D.C.: Government Printing Office, 2000). There is also a *Healthy People 2010*.

2. There are exceptions. For example, Louise Walter, Karla Lindquist, and Kenneth Covinsky published an article entitled "Relationship between Health Status and Use of Screening Mammography and Papanicolaou Smears Among Women Older Than 70 Years of Age," *Annals of Internal Medicine,* 140 (2004): 681–688, which was picked up by the Boston Globe in a series of articles about screening in their health section on May 4, 2004.

3. U.S. Preventive Services Task Force, "Screening for Prostate Cancer: Recommendations and Rationale." Updated 2003. The USPSTF does not recommend PSA screening for anyone, but says that if it is useful at all, it would most likely be so in men aged 50–70. See also J. W. Feighter, "Screening for Prostate Cancer," Canadian Task Force on the Periodic Health Examination, *Canadian Guide to Clinical Preventive Health Care* (Ottawa, 1994), pp. 812–823.

4. Laurence Beck, "Periodic Health Examination and Screening Tests in Adults," *Hospital Practice* (Office Edition), 34 (1999): 117–118, 121–122, 124–126.

5. L. Breslow and A. R. Somers, "The Lifetime Health-Monitoring Program: A Practical Approach to Preventive Medicine," *New England Journal of Medicine*, 296 (1977): 601.

6. Sylvia Oboler, Allan Prochazka, Ralph Gonzales, Stanley Xu, and Robert Anderson, "Public Expectations and Attitudes for Annual Physical Examinations and Testing," *Annals of Internal Medicine*, 136 (2002): 652–659.

7. Christine Laine, "The Annual Physical Examination: Needless Ritual or Necessary Routine?" *Annals of Internal Medicine*, 136 (2002): 701–703.

8. Even randomized studies cannot answer the question of whether the new treatment is preferable to the existing treatment (when there is one) unless the two approaches are compared to each other. The Food and Drug Administration currently requires that new medications be compared to a placebo rather than to the available medication, which raises yet another obstacle to determining the best treatment. For a discussion of drug companies, see Marcia Angell, *The Truth About the Drug Companies: How They Deceive Us and What to Do About It* (N.Y.: Random House, 2004).

9. J. Bruce Mosely, Kimberly O'Malley, Nancy Petersen, et al., "A Controlled Trial of Arthroscopic Surgery for Osteoarthritis of the Knee," *New England Journal of Medicine*, 347 (2002): 81–88.

10. David Felson and Joseph Buckwalter, "Debridement and Lavage for Osteoarthritis of the Knee," *New England Journal of Medicine*, 347 (2002): 132–133.

11. Stephen Hulley, Deborah Grady, Trudy Bush, et al., "Randomized Trial

of Estrogen plus Progestin as Secondary Prevention of Coronary Heart Disease in Postmenopausal Women. Heart and Estrogen/Progestin Replacement Study (HERS) Research Group," *Journal of the American Medical Association*, 280 (1998): 605–613; Writing Group for the Women's Health Initiative Investigators, "Risks and Benefits of Estrogen Plus Progestin in Healthy Postmenopausal Women: Principal Results from the Women's Health Initiative Randomized Controlled Trial," *Journal of the American Medical Association*, 288 (2002): 321–333; Christine Laine, "Post-Menopausal Hormone Replacement Therapy: How Could We Have Been So Wrong?" *Annals of Internal Medicine*, 137 (2002): 290.

12. The Prostate Cancer Outcomes Study found that 42 percent of men reported occasional leakage. Impotence after surgery depended on age, with 100 percent of men in their seventies reporting impotence. Nerve-sparing surgery is better but is not advocated in patients with high PSA scores, large tumors, and higher-grade tumors (that is, more microscopically malignant). See Joanna Madalinska, Marie-Louise Essink-Bot, Harry de Koning, et al., "Health-related Quality-of-Life Effects of Radical Prostatectomy and Primary Radiotherapy for Screen-Detected or Clinically Diagnosed Local Prostate Cancer," *Journal of Clinical Oncology*, 29 (2001): 1619–1628.

13. Lars Holmberg, Anna Bill-Axelson, Fred Helgesen, et al., "A Randomized Trial Comparing Radical Prostatectomy with Watchful Waiting in Early Prostate Cancer," *New England Journal of Medicine*, 347 (2002): 781–789.

14. Lisa Kowalcyzk, "Full-body Disagreement," *Boston Globe*, June 28, 2002.

15. Ibid.

16. BBC Home Page, "US Doctors Offer Full Body Scan," BBC News, January 2, 2001.

17. Kenneth Chu, Charles Smart, and Robert Tarone, "Analysis of Breast Cancer Mortality and Stage Distribution by Age for the Health Insurance Plan Clinical Trial," *Journal of the National Cancer Institute*, 80 (1988): 1125–1132; Douglas Rex, David Johnson, David Lieberman, et al., "Colorectal Cancer Prevention 2000: Screening Recommendations of the American College of Gastroenterology," *American Journal of Gastroenterology*, 95 (2000): 868–877.

18. The leading study was the Hypertension Detection and Follow-Up Program Cooperative Group, which presented its "Five-Year Findings of the Hypertension Detection and Follow-Up Program" in the *Journal of the American Medical Association* in 1979 (vol. 242: 2562–2571). All-cause mortality was lower in patients whose hypertension was treated, principally as a result of a decrease in heart attacks and strokes.

19. SHEP Cooperative Research Group, "Prevention of Stroke by Antihypertensive Drug Treatment in Older Persons with Isolated Systolic Hypertension: Final Results of the Systolic Hypertension in the Elderly Program," *Journal of the American Medical Association,* 265 (1991): 3255–3264. And similar findings had already been reported by the Europeans: see A. Amery, P. Brixko, D. Clement, et al., "Mortality and Morbidity Results from the European Working Party on High Blood Pressure in the Elderly Trial," *Lancet,* 1, 8442 (1985): 1349–1354.

20. Kenneth Manton and James Vaupel, "Survival After the Age of 80 in the United States, Sweden, France, England, and Japan," *New England Journal of Medicine,* 333 (1995): 1232–1235.

21. This kind of schema is laid out nicely for cancer screening by Louise Walter and Kenneth Covinsky in their article, "Cancer Screening in Elderly Patients: A Framework for Individualized Decision Making," *Journal of the American Medical Association,* 285 (2001): 2750–2756.

22. Edward Hannan, Jay Magaziner, Jason Wang, et al., "Mortality and Locomotion 6 Months after Hospitalization for Hip Fracture: Risk Factors and Risk-Adjusted Hospital Outcomes," *Journal of the American Medical Association,* 285 (2001): 2736–2742.

23. A. S. Robbins, L. Z. Rubenstein, K. R. Josephson, et al., "Prediction of Falls Among Elderly People: Results of Two Population-Based Studies," *Archives of Internal Medicine,* 149 (1989): 1628–1633. This study is old, but still pertinent. A practice guideline for physicians, indicating how to screen for falls and then how to do a falls evaluation, was put together jointly by the American Geriatrics Society, the British Geriatrics Society, and the American Academy of Orthopaedic Surgeons' Panel on Falls Prevention: "Guidelines for the Prevention of Falls in Older Persons," *Journal of the American Geriatric Society,* 49 (2001): 664–672.

24. S. Wolf, H. Barnhart, N. Kutner, et al., "Reducing Fractures and Falls in

Older Persons: An Investigation of Tai Chi and Computerized Balance Training," *Journal of the American Geriatric Society,* 44 (1996): 489–497. And see the recent review by M. E. Tinetti, "Clinical Practice: Preventing Falls in Elderly Persons," *New England Journal of Medicine,* 348 (2003): 42–49, where several interesting studies are cited. In one, tapering psychotropic medications over a 14-week period led to a 33 percent reduction in the risk of falls. In another, a home evaluation by an occupational therapist to identify risks such as throw rugs and poor lighting decreased the risk of falls by 20 percent. More effective than any single intervention are combination strategies that evaluate the home *and* review medications *and* prescribe exercise programs.

25.   P. D. Ross, "Osteoporosis: Frequency, Consequences, and Risk Factors," *Archives of Internal Medicine,* 156 (1996): 1399–1411.

26.   P. Kannus, J. Patikkari, S. Niemi, et al., "Prevention of Hip Fracture in Elderly People with Use of a Hip Protector," *New England Journal of Medicine,* 343 (2000): 1506–1513.

27.   Much of the groundbreaking work in this area is by Lisa Berkman and her colleagues. A study that looks at this phenomenon after a heart attack is L. Berkman, L. Leo-Summers, and R. Horwitz, "Emotional Support and Survival After Myocardial Infarction: A Prospective, Population-Based Study of the Elderly," *Annals of Internal Medicine,* 117 (1992): 1003–1009.

28.   A study of disability rates after hospitalization for hip fracture, stroke, or heart attack as a function of social support is V. Wilcox, S. Kash, and L. Berkman, "Social Support and Physical Disability in Older People After Hospitalization: A Prospective Study," *Health Psychology,* 13 (1994): 170–179.

29.   S. S. Bassuk, T. A. Glass, and L. F. Berkman, "Social Disengagement and Incident Cognitive Decline in Community-Dwelling Elderly Persons," *Annals of Internal Medicine,* 131 (1999): 165–173.

2. When Less Is More

1.   There is no uniformly agreed-upon definition of frailty. It's one of those conditions where you know it if you see it. One of the leading hypotheses is that it is a syndrome characterized by weakness and poor

nutritional status. In effect, it is a wasting syndrome, like AIDS or cancer-induced cachexia. This is the view propounded by L. Fried, C. Tazen, J. Walson, et al., "Frailty in Older Adults: Evidence for a Phenotype," *Gerontology,* 56 (2001): 146–157. I have argued, by contrast, for the vulnerability model of frailty: it is a condition in which any sort of provocation, whether a physical or emotional stress, can tip a person into illness. See Muriel Gillick, "Pinning Down Frailty," *Journal of Gerontology Series A: Biological and Medical Sciences,* 56A (2001): M134–M135.

2. Thomas Lee and Lee Goldman, "Evaluation of the Patient with Acute Chest Pain," *New England Journal of Medicine,* 342 (2000): 1187–1195. The CPK-MB is very specific for cardiac tissue and was the preferred marker for many years. It begins to rise 3–6 hours after the onset of a myocardial infarction, and is not elevated in all patients until 12 hours have passed. If the initial test is normal and the EKG is not diagnostic and the clinical suspicion remains high (which was not the case with my patient), then follow-up testing over the next 24 hours is indicated.

3. S. Inouye, S. Bogardus, P. Charpentier, et al., "A Multi-Component Intervention to Prevent Delirium in Hospitalized Older Patients," *New England Journal of Medicine,* 340 (1999): 669–676; J. Fitzgerald and R. Dittus, "Institutionalized Patients with Hip Fractures: Characteristics Associated with Returning to Community Dwelling," *Journal of General Internal Medicine,* 5 (1990): 298–303. These authors found that patients who were discharged to a skilled nursing facility for rehabilitation after hospitalization for a hip fracture were more likely to return to their homes if they walked while in the hospital.

4. J. L. Thistle, P. A. Cleary, J. M. Lachin, et al., "The Natural History of Cholelithiasis: The Natural Cooperative Gallstone Study," *Annals of Internal Medicine,* 201 (1984): 171–175.

5. The SUPPORT Principal Investigators, "A Controlled Trial to Improve Care for Seriously Ill Hospitalized Patients: The Study to Understand Prognoses and Preferences for Care (SUPPORT)," *Journal of the American Medical Association,* 274 (1995): 1591–1598.

6. A classic study looked at the importance of patient preference in selecting between two treatments: B. McNeil, R. Weichselbaum, and S. Pauker, "Speech and Survival: Tradeoffs between Quality and Quantity

of Life in Laryngeal Cancer," *New England Journal of Medicine,* 305 (1981): 1982–1987.

7. T. Fried, E. Bradley, V. Towle, and H. Allore, "Understanding the Treatment Preferences of Seriously Ill Patients," *New England Journal of Medicine,* 346 (2002): 1061–1066.

8. See Eric Cassell, *The Nature of Suffering and the Goals of Medicine* (New York: Oxford University Press, 1991).

9. The Health Care Financing Administration released hospital mortality statistics to help consumers select a hospital starting in 1986. Bruce Vladeck, head of HCFA, discontinued the practice in 1993 on the grounds that it did not in fact affect patient choice.

10. Muriel Gillick, "Doing the Right Thing: Quality Assurance in the Elderly," *Journal of the American Geriatrics Society,* 42 (1994): 1024–1026. When I was doing the final work on this chapter, an article was published which demonstrated very dramatically what can happen when "guidelines" fail to consider how sick a person is and what his preferences are. See Louise Walter, Natalie Davidowitz, Paul Heineken, and Kenneth Covinsky, "Pitfalls of Converting Practice Guidelines into Quality Measures: Lessons Learned from a VA Performance Measure," *Journal of the American Medical Association,* 291 (2004): 2466–2470. The authors found that physicians and hospitals were considered to be providing substandard care if they failed to order screening tests for colorectal cancer, even if the patients in question were unlikely to benefit from the screening or stated clearly that they didn't want the test.

11. Confusion after coronary artery bypass surgery is commonplace. The long-term consequences are more controversial. See M. Newman, J. Kirchner, B. Phillips-Bute, et al., "Longitudinal Assessment of Neurocognitive Functioning After Coronary-Artery Bypass Surgery," *New England Journal of Medicine,* 344 (2001): 395–412; in their carefully done study, they reported that 53 percent of patients undergoing bypass surgery had cognitive decline at the time of discharge from the hospital, 36 percent had decline at 6 weeks, 24 percent at 6 months. Interestingly, the rate of cognitive impairment at 5 years was 42 percent, with abnormal cognitive function at discharge from the hospital a predictor of long-term abnormalities.

12. Morphine works by decreasing anxiety and the work of breathing. This in turn causes a decrease in the outpouring of epinephrine-like substances that is normally triggered by anxiety. The diminution in this "central sympathetic outflow" causes the arteries and veins to relax.

13. Terminal sedation is a somewhat controversial practice sometimes used for treatment of excruciating symptoms in a dying patient that are refractory to conventional means. It involves giving sedation sufficient to induce unconsciousness and withholding artificial nutrition and hydration to allow death to occur.

14. Current thinking is that a heart attack is often due to ruptured plaque that causes an acute narrowing or obstruction of a blood vessel, not to gradual narrowing from atherosclerosis as was previously believed.

15. See T. Bodenheim, E. Wagner, and K. Grumbach, "Improving Primary Care for Patients with Chronic Illness: The Chronic Care Mode. Part 2," *Journal of the American Medical Association*, 288 (2002): 1909–1914.

16. For a more extensive discussion of the meaning and implications of frailty, see my book entitled *Lifelines: Living Longer, Growing Frail, Taking Heart* (New York: Norton, 2001).

17. The decline was first noted when the period 1968–1976 was studied: L. Goldman and E. Cook, "The Decline in Ischemic Heart Disease Mortality Rates," *Annals of Internal Medicine*, 101 (1984): 825–836. The death rate from ischemic heart disease fell 21 percent between 1968 and 1976, with more than half of the decline attributable to life-style changes. The analysis was continued in M. Hunink, L. Goldman, and A. Tosteson, "The Recent Decline in Mortality from Coronary Heart Disease, 1980–1990," *Journal of the American Medical Association*, 277 (1997): 535–542. These authors found that the incidence (new cases per year) was falling 1 percent each year, which it had done continuously for three decades, and mortality was falling between 2 and 4 percent per year.

18. The father of chronic disease management is Edward Wagner. He defines this approach as involving "planned regular interactions with caregivers," focusing on the prevention of exacerbations and complications. Key features are patient self-management, patient education,

and feedback to nurse practitioners who work together with physicians. Edward Wagner, "Chronic Disease Management: What Will It Take to Improve Care for Chronic Illness?" *Effective Clinical Practice,* 1 (1998): 2–4.

19. The data come from the Agency on Health Quality Research, Healthcare Costs and Utilization Project, and are cited in a white paper by ITAA called "Chronic Care Improvement: How Medicare Transformation Can Save Lives, Save Money, and Stimulate an Emerging Technology Industry" (Arlington, Va., May 2004). See also J. Croft, W. Giles, R. Pollard, et al., "Heart Failure Survival Among Older Adults in the United States," *Archives of Internal Medicine,* 159 (1999): 505–510.

20. S. Stewart, S. Pearson, and J. Horowitz, "Effects of a Home-Based Intervention among Patients with Congestive Heart Failure Discharged from Acute Hospital," *Archives of Internal Medicine,* 158 (1998): 1067–1072; S. Stewart, A. Vanderbrock, S. Pearson, and J. Horowitz, "Prolonged Beneficial Effects of a Home-Based Intervention on Unplanned Readmissions and Mortality Among Patients with Congestive Heart Failure," *Archives of Internal Medicine,* 159 (1999): 257–261.

21. There have now been multiple studies of chronic disease management for heart failure patients. A review of the best of these studies is F. McAlister, F. Lawson, K. Teo, and P. Armstrong, "A Systematic Review of Randomized Trials of Disease Management Programs in Heart Failure," *American Journal of Medicine,* 110 (2001): 378–384. A total of eleven studies were identified, involving 2,067 patients. Cost savings were found in all but one, and the risk of hospitalization was markedly decreased with disease management.

22. S. J. Wilson, P. S. Wells, M. J. Kovacs, et al., "Comparing the Quality of Oral Anticoagulant Management by Anticoagulation Clinics and by Family Physicians: A Randomised Controlled Trial," *Canadian Medical Association Journal,* 169 (2003): 293–298.

23. J. Lafata, S. Martin, S. Kaatz, and R. Ward, "The Cost Effectiveness of Different Management Strategies for Patients on Chronic Warfarin Therapy," *Journal of General Internal Medicine,* 15 (2000): 31–37. Anticoagulation clinics were associated with a decrease in the bleeding rate of 2/1000 compared to usual care, and self-monitoring led to a further 0.8/1000 decrease in bleeding. Both clinics and self-monitoring were

cheaper than physician monitoring. See also a small randomized trial: M. E. Cromheecke, M. Levi, L. Colly, et al., "Oral Anticoagulation Self-Management and Management by a Specialist Anticoagulation Clinic: A Randomised Cross-Over Comparison," *Lancet*, 356 (2000): 97–102. In this study, the medication was in the therapeutic range 55 percent of the time with self-management and 49 percent of the time with clinic management.

24. N. Naylor, D. Brooten, R. Campbell, et al., "Comprehensive Discharge Planning and Home Follow-up of Hospitalized Elders: A Randomized Clinical Trial," *Journal of the American Medical Association*, 281 (1999): 613–620. In this study, advance practice nurses monitored high-risk patients over age 75, which resulted in a fall in the rate of readmission to the hospital (measured at 6 months after the initial discharge to home) from 37 percent to 20 percent.

25. The Medicare Modernization Act of 2003 commits the Centers for Medicare and Medicaid Services, which administers the Medicare program, to fund several demonstration programs for chronically ill patients. It is particularly interested in disease management programs targeting Medicare beneficiaries with congestive heart failure, diabetes, and chronic obstructive pulmonary disease.

3. Doing the Right Thing Near the End

1. Michael Bliss, *William Osler: A Life in Medicine* (New York: Oxford University Press, 1999). What Osler actually said was "pneumonia is the captain of the men of death." He also said, in an address given at Johns Hopkins University when he himself was 56, that men over age 60 were entirely useless.

2. National Conference of Catholic Bishops, "Ethical and Religious Directives for Catholic Health Care Services, Fourth Edition" (Washington, D.C.: U.S. Catholic Conference, 2001). In March of 2004, Pope John Paul II elaborated on this matter. In speaking to a congress of physicians and ethicists, he stated that artificial nutrition and hydration are required for individuals in a persistent vegetative state. Perhaps he recognized that there is no direct burden to a patient in a vegetative state from artificial nutrition or from anything else, since the

individual cannot experience anything. What he said was that in this situation, "administration of food and water, even when provided by artificial means, always represents a natural means of preserving life, not a medical act," and he added that providing nutrition and hydration is "in principle, ordinary and proportionate, and as such, morally obligatory." Quoted in "Allowing to Die II," *Commonweal* Magazine, April 23, 2004, p. 8.

3. Fred Friedman, "The Chronic Vegetative Patient: A Torah Perspective," *Journal of Halacha and Contemporary Society,* 26 (1993): 88–109.

4. Moshe Tendler, *Responsa of Rav Moshe Feinstein, Col. 1: Care of the Critically Ill* (Hoboken, N.J.: KTAV Publishing House, 1996).

5. S. J. Youngner, "Who Defines Futility?" *Journal of the American Medical Association,* 260 (1988): 2094–2095.

6. L. J. Schneiderman, N. S. Jecker, and A. R. Jonsen, "Medical Futility: Its Meaning and Ethical Implications," *Annals of Internal Medicine,* 113 (1990): 949–954.

7. Some organizations have gone to extremes in seeking to define futility. The American Heart Association, for example, in attempting to state when CPR did not have to be performed because it would with certainty be unsuccessful, indicated that resuscitation did not have to be done in cases of decapitation. American Heart Association, "Standards and Guidelines for Cardiopulmonary Resuscitation (CPR) and Emergency Cardiac Care (ECC): Part VIII, Medicolegal Considerations and Recommendations," *Journal of the American Medical Association,* 255 (1986): 2979–2984.

8. S. H. Miles, "Informed Demand for 'Non-Beneficial' Medical Treatment," *New England Journal of Medicine,* 325 (1991): 512–515.

9. R. E. Cranford, "Helga Wanglie's Ventilator," *Hastings Center Report,* 21 (1991): 23–24.

10. American Medical Association, "Medical Futility in End-of-Life Care: Report of the Council on Ethical and Judicial Affairs," *Journal of the American Medical Association,* 211 (1999): 939–941; P. R. Helft, M. Siegler, and J. Lantos, "The Rise and Fall of the Futility Movement," *New England Journal of Medicine,* 343 (2000): 293–296.

11. R. S. Morrison and A. L. Siu, "Survival in End-Stage Dementia Following Acute Illness," *Journal of the American Medical Association,* 284 (2000): 47–52.

12. This number is obtained by extrapolating from two different studies. One study found that 22 percent of ICU resources are devoted to what the authors called potentially ineffective care (in-hospital death or death within 100 days of hospital discharge and total hospital costs over the 90th percentile): D. J. Cher and L. A. Lenert, "Method of Medicare Reimbursement and the Rate of Potentially Ineffective Care of Critically Ill Patients," *Journal of the American Medical Association,* 278 (1997): 1001–1007. A second study estimated that ICU costs are 20 percent of total hospital costs, or $70 billion in 1995: J. Luce and G. Rubenfeld, "Can Health Care Costs Be Reduced by Limiting Intensive Care at the End of Life?" *American Journal of Respiratory Critical Care Medicine,* 165 (2002): 750–754. 22 percent of $70 billion is $15.46 billion.

13. Multi-Society Task Force on Medical Aspects of the Persistent Vegetative State: First of Two Parts. *New England Journal of Medicine,* 330 (1994): 1499–1508.

14. K. J. Fabiszewski, B. Volicer, and L. Volicer, "Effect of Antibiotic Treatment on Outcome of Fever in Institutionalized Alzheimer Patients," *Journal of the American Medical Association,* 263 (1990): 3168–3172.

15. D. B. Waisel and R. D. Truog, "The Cardiopulmonary Resuscitation–Not-Indicated Order: Futility Revisited," *Annals of Internal Medicine,* 122 (1995): 304–308. This article reviews four sample CPR-not-indicated policies from the Allegheny General Hospital in Pittsburgh, Pennsylvania, the Veterans Affairs Medical Center in Seattle, Washington, the Beth Israel Hospital in Boston, Massachusetts, and the Johns Hopkins Hospital in Baltimore, Maryland. The Beth Israel Hospital policy says the circumstances are as follows: "The patient is dying with no chance of recovery or there is no reasonable likelihood that CPR efforts would be successful in restoring cardiac and pulmonary function . . . and the proposed treatment would increase or prolong the patient's suffering."

16. G. Kolata, "Case of Catherine Gilgunn. Court Ruling Limits Rights of Patients: Care Deemed Futile May Be Withheld," *New York Times,* April 22, 1995, p. 6.

17. See David Orentlicher, *Matters of Life and Death* (Princeton, N.J.: Princeton University Press, 2001), pp. 164–166.

18. B. Spielman, "Community Futility Policies: The Illusion of Consen-

sus?" In H. Zucker and M. Zucker, eds., *Medical Futility: A Critical Evaluation of Treatment Decisions* (New York: Cambridge University Press, 1997), pp. 168–178.

19. D. J. Murphy and E. Barbour, "GUIDe (Guidelines for the Use of Intensive Care in Denver): A Community Effort to Define Futile and Inappropriate Care," *New Horizons*, 2 (1994): 326–331.

20. A. Halevy and B. A. Brody, "A Multi-Institution Collaborative Policy on Medical Futility," *Journal of the American Medical Association*, 276 (1996): 571–574.

21. A handful of interested ethicists put together a conference with 74 participants (physicians, lawyers, judges, nurses, social workers, members of the clergy, and community representatives) drawn from 39 hospitals in California. They represented academic medical centers, community hospitals, HMOs, and religiously affiliated health care facilities throughout California. In a one-day conference in San Diego, they reviewed cases and hospital futility policies and concluded that hospitals should establish a clear process for resolving disputes over futility. See L. J. Schneiderman and A. M. Capron, "How Can Hospital Futility Policies Contribute to Establishing Standards of Practice?" *Cambridge Quarterly of Healthcare Ethics*, 9 (2000): 524–531. See also Health Ethics Committee of the Health Council of South Florida, Inc., *The Medical Futility Guidelines of South Florida*, February 2000 *(www .healthcouncil.org)*.

22. J. R. Curtis, D. D. Park, M. R. Krone, and R. A. Pearlman, "Use of the Medical Futility Rationale in Do-Not-Attempt-Resuscitation Orders," *Journal of the American Medical Association*, 273 (1995): 124–128. The authors of this study interviewed 145 hospital physicians who had written "DNAR" orders for hospitalized patients, including 91 for whom the rationale for the order was futility. They found that in the patients where "quantitative" futility applied (that is, there was a low probability of success), the physicians estimated the actual likelihood of survival to discharge as varying from 0–75 percent, with 32 percent predicting the likelihood of survival to be greater than 5 percent. For those patients in whom "qualitative" futility applied (that is, there would be poor quality of life if CPR were performed), the physicians made the judgment about futility without talking to the patients.

23. Stephen Toulmin commented on his experience as a staff member on a major government commission: "When the eleven individual commissioners asked themselves what 'principles' underlay and supposedly justified their adhesion to the consensus, each of them answered in his or her own way: the Catholics appealed to Catholic principles, the humanists to humanist principles, and so on. They could agree; they could agree what they were agreeing about; but, apparently, they could not agree why they agreed with it." See S. Toulmin, "The Tyranny of Principles," *Hastings Center Report,* 11 (1981): 31–39.

24. A model for achieving agreement that has been reasonably effective is the Consensus Conference sponsored by the National Institutes of Health. Approaches to osteoporosis screening or geriatric assessment have been reviewed by these conferences, with medical experts testifying as to their efficacy. A broad spectrum of the population is invited to attend and ask questions, which has led to the issuance of practical, cogent guidelines with a wide base of support.

25. Oregon is the only state in the United States where physician-assisted suicide is legal. However, it has been the subject of referenda in several other states and under discussion in the state legislatures of still others. Physician-assisted suicide became legal in Oregon in 1997 and has been legal in the Netherlands since 2003, though it was quasi-legal long before that. As a result, researchers have had the opportunity to study who requests PAS and why, and who actually takes the pills once a prescription is written. The number-one reason for wanting PAS is not pain, not unbearable suffering, and not fear of being a burden to one's family. The principal reason why dying patients request phenobarbital, according to their families, is that they fear loss of autonomy and loss of control of their bodily function. Physical suffering is a distant third, and concern about being a burden to their families is the next most commonly expressed concern. These findings, which are confined to the relatively homogenous populations of Oregon and Holland, are mirrored in national polls of cancer patients and others near the end of life. When asked whether PAS should be legal, the majority of those surveyed say it should. Most do not contemplate actually availing themselves of the opportunity to end their lives, but say that they want to be able to control the circumstances of their death.

26. A. Chin, K. Hedberg, G. Higginson, and D. Fleming, "Legalized Physician-Assisted Suicide in Oregon—the First Year's Experience," *New England Journal of Medicine*, 340 (1999): 577–583; A. Sullivan, K. Hedberg, and D. Fleming, "Legalized Physician-Assisted Suicide in Oregon—the Second Year," *New England Journal of Medicine*, 342 (2000): 598–604. In 1999, 26 of the 33 patients who received a prescription for lethal medications committed suicide. Five died from their underlying disease, and two were alive at the end of the year.

27. P. Singer, D. Martin, and M. Kelner, "Quality End-of-Life Care: Patients' Perspectives," *Journal of the American Medical Association*, 281 (1999): 163–168. This was a qualitative face-to-face interview study of patients undergoing dialysis, living in a long-term care facility, or suffering from HIV infection. The authors identified five areas of concern for quality of life. Patients said they wanted to receive adequate pain and symptom management, they wanted to avoid prolongation of dying, they wanted to achieve a sense of control, they did not want to be a burden, and they wanted to strengthen their relationships with those they loved.

28. In this case, giving medication to "end it all" technically would have been euthanasia rather than physician-assisted suicide, since Mr. Robinson was no longer able to understand the issues and request the means to end his life. The patient's family sought to end his life because they felt he would have regarded his state of limited autonomy as unendurable.

29. Cicely Saunders, "A Personal Therapeutic Journey," *British Medical Journal*, 313 (1996): 1599–1601.

30. Quoted in Cancer Source, "Ask Dr. Cicely Saunders." Interview, August 28, 2001, *www.cancersource.com*.

31. "Dying with dignity" has become a trite phrase. Moreover, dignity is sometimes hard to achieve, as Sherwin Nuland points out in *How We Die* (New York: Knopf, 1994). Ira Byock, a leader in the palliative care field, advocates instead that we speak of "dying well." The phrase is the title of his book, *Dying Well* (New York: Riverside Books, 1998).

32. L. Ganzini, H. Nelson, T. Schmidt, et al., "Physicians' Experience with the Oregon Death with Dignity Act," *New England Journal of Medicine*, 302 (2000): 557–563.

4. The Trouble with Medicare

1. An opinion poll undertaken by the Kaiser Family Foundation together with the Harvard School of Public Health found that 74 percent of those polled thought Medicare did a good job. Among those polled who were under 65 years of age, only 34 percent knew that Medicare doesn't pay for long-term care. Kaiser Family Foundation/Harvard School of Public Health National Survey on Medicare, Kaiser Family Foundation, Washington, D.C., October 20, 1998 *(http://www.kff.org/medicare/1442-reform_pr.cfm).*

2. The full name is actually the Medicare Prescription Drug, Improvement, and Modernization Act, P.L. 108-173. The act contains a number of provisions in addition to coverage for prescription drugs, such as incentives to prepaid health plans to enroll seniors.

3. M. Moon, "Medicare: Health Policy 2001," *New England Journal of Medicine,* 344 (2001): 928–931. Currently, Medicare beneficiaries pay ⁱⁿᵗ ᶜ ᵗ :ket each year for health care, not count-resents 20 percent of their income, up l1 percent shortly after Medicare was in-

s on an article I wrote with a colleague in ell, "A Framework for Meaningful Medi-g and Social Policy, 16 (2004): 1–12.
D. Witt, "Effectiveness and Economic Im-am for Outpatient Management of Acute Group Model Health Maintenance Orga-l Medicine, 160 (2000): 2926–2932.
eep vein thrombophlebitis" in 2005 is n of hospitalization is 4.5 days, as reported for Medical Care, "Physician Documenta-ive Payment System Reimbursement," Jan-

n of the Medicare Modernization Act is Kaiser Family Foundation, "Medicare Fact cff.org. The standard benefit, in effect as of tients paying the first $250 in drug costs, 25 percent of yearly drug costs between $250 and $2250, and 100 percent of yearly drug costs between $2250 and $5100 (informally known as the "hole in the doughnut"). After patients have paid $3600 out of pocket (for $5100 worth of medications), they pay approximately 5 percent of any additional expenditures.

8. It is precisely this sort of concern that led me to propose the creation of special geriatric hospitals. See M. R. Gillick, "Do We Need to Create Geriatric Hospitals?" *Journal of the American Geriatrics Society,* 50 (2002): 174–177.

9. See M. Lachs and H. Ruchlin, "Is Managed Care Good or Bad for Geriatric Medicine?" *Journal of the American Geriatric Society,* 45 (1997): 1123–1127.

10. J. L. Ahronheim, R. S. Morrison, S. A. Baskin, et al., "Treatment of the Dying in the Acute Care Hospital: Advanced Dementia and Metastatic Cancer," *Archives of Internal Medicine,* 156 (1996): 2094–2100.

11. Last Acts, "Means to a Better End: A Report on Dying in America Today," November 2002. Available at *http://www.rwjf.org/files/publications/other/meansbetterend.pdf.*

12. For many years the National Hospice and Palliative Care Organization has administered a family satisfaction survey to families after the death of a loved one. More than 250 hospices use the instrument. It includes questions such as: "Based on your experience, would you recommend hospice to others?" to which between 95 and 99 percent of those surveyed reply yes. S. Connor, J. Teno, C. Spence, and N. Smith, "Family Evaluation of Hospice Care," *Journal of Pain and Symptom Management,* 30 (2005): 9–17.

13. J. Lynn and J. H. Forlini, "Serious and Complex Illness in Quality Improvement and Policy Reform for End-of-Life Care," *Journal of General Internal Medicine,* 16, no. 5 (2001): 315–319.

14. MedPAC Report to Congress, "Hospice Care in Medicare: Recent Trends and a Review of the Issues," June 4, 2004. *www.medpac.gov/publications/congressional_reports/June04_ch6.pdf,* accessed June 10, 2005.

15. Medicare defines as "homebound" someone who requires considerable effort and assistance to leave home, and who intermittently needs care. In practice, the interpretation varies. The most generous inter-

pretation is that a person is homebound if he has an illness that restricts his ability to leave home except with the assistance of a supportive device, special transport, or another person.

16. The exact distribution of the pie varies over time, but recent statistics suggest that Medicaid pays 46 percent of all nursing home costs, Medicare pays 12 percent, private long-term care insurance covers 12 percent, other government payors account for 2 percent (such as the Veterans Administration), and 28 percent is paid out of pocket by the elderly. Kaiser Commission on Medicare and the Uninsured, "Medicaid and Long-Term Care," March 2005.

17. T. J. Mattimore, N. S. Wenger, N. A. Desbiens, et al., "Surrogate and Physician Understanding of Patients' Preferences for Living Permanently in a Nursing Home," *Journal of the American Geriatrics Society,* 45 (1997): 818–824.

18. The MetLife Market Survey of Nursing Home and Home Care Costs, September 2004. *http://www.metlife.com/WPSAssets/165828858111060 64631V1FNursing%20Home%20Home%.*

19. The rates vary depending on geography. The numbers cited here are average private pay rates, as determined from a survey done by the State of Connecticut, Office of Policy and Management, in January 2004 *(www.opm.state.ct.us/pdpd4/ltc/consumer/nhrate.htm).*

20. S. L. Mitchell, "Financial Incentives to Place Feeding Tubes in Nursing Home Residents with Advanced Dementia," *Journal of the American Geriatrics Society,* 51 (2003): 129–131; S. Mitchell, J. Buchanan, S. Littlehale, and M. Hamel, "Tube-Feeding Versus Hand-Feeding Nursing Home Residents with Advanced Dementia: A Cost Comparison," *Journal of the American Medical Directors Association,* 4 (2003): 27–33.

21. MedPAC Report to Congress, "Hospice Care in Medicare." The percentage of Medicare "decedents" who used hospice care tripled between 1992 and 2000. But the duration of enrollment continues to decline.

22. National PACE Association, *www.npaonline.org.*

23. Nora Super, "Medicare's Chronic Care Improvement Pilot Program: What Is Its Potential?" Health Policy Forum Issue Brief no. 797, May 10, 2004,*www.nhpf.03/pdfs_ib/IB797_ChronicCare.pdf.* The pilot pro-

gram to improve chronic care management will focus on patients with one of three conditions: congestive heart failure, diabetes, or chronic lung disease.

24. See my article "Medicare Coverage for Technological Innovations: Time for New Criteria?" *New England Journal of Medicine,* 350 (2004): 2199–2203.

25. E. Rose, A. Gelihns, A. Moskowitz, et al., "Long-term Use of a Left Ventricular Assist Device for End-stage Heart Failure," *New England Journal of Medicine,* 345 (2003): 1435–1443. The Centers for Medicare and Medicaid Services agreed to pay for this device in selected Medicare patients on October 1, 2003. Interestingly, the device costs $65,000 and the total hospital charges run to about $200,000, although Medicare has so far only agreed to pay about $70,000 plus physician fees, which are billed separately.

26. National Emphysema Treatment Trial Research Group, "A Randomized Trial Comparing Lung-Volume–Reduction Surgery with Medical Surgery in Severe Emphysema," *New England Journal of Medicine,* 348 (2003): 2059–2073. This technology was approved for Medicare reimbursement in August 2003.

27. See Marilyn J. Field and Christine K. Cassel, eds., *Approaching Death: Improving Care at the End of Life* (Washington, D.C.: National Academy Press, 1997), for a description of these trajectories. The per diem rate paid to hospice for "routine" home care in 2005 was $122.98.

28. The Centers for Medicare and Medicaid Services provides information to the general public about these choices through its brochure, revised annually: "Medicare and You" (2006). This is available on the CMS Web site at *www.medicare.gov/publications/pubs/pdf/10050.pdf.*

29. As mentioned in Chapter 3, physicians discuss diagnosis but rarely prognosis with their cancer patients (E. B. Lamont and N. A. Christakis, "Prognostic Disclosures to Patients with Cancer Near the End of Life," *Annals of Internal Medicine,* 134 (2001): 1096–1105). They rarely discuss the prognosis of other diseases, such as congestive heart failure or advanced liver disease (R. W. Wachter, J. M. Luce, N. Hearst, and B. Lo, "Decisions about Resuscitation: Inequities Among Patients with Different Diseases but Similar Prognoses," *Annals of Internal Medicine,* 111 (1989) 525–532). If physicians do not discuss prognosis in pa-

tients with a single disease, they are even less likely to do so with patients who have multiple interacting conditions.

30. Concerns have been raised about whether providing different benefit packages to patients on the basis of their underlying health status violates the Americans with Disabilities Act. The ADA prohibits discrimination against people with disabilities in access to public insurance programs and to physician services. However, the courts have concluded that "equal benefits" is not the same as "equivalent benefits." Because healthy people are different in important ways from disabled people, and by inference frail people are different from those who are robust or who are dying, they may need to be treated differently in order to be treated as equals. The Supreme Court has observed that "sometimes the greatest discrimination can lie in treating things that are different as though they were exactly alike," as reported by David Orentlicher in his article "Rationing and the Americans with Disabilities Act," *Journal of the American Medical Association*, 271 (1994): 308–314. Clearly, there will be more legal challenges to the three benefit packages approach if they are not freely chosen by beneficiaries.

31. Many instruments exist for assessing these domains. The most commonly used are the Charlson index for disease burden, the Katz ADL index for function, and the Folstein Mini-mental state examination for cognitive function.

32. Social Security Act, sec. 1862[a][1], amended 1965.

33. Medically Necessary Services, *www.medicarerights.org*.

5. Is a Nursing Home in Your Future?

1. B. C. Spillman and J. Lubitz, "New Estimates of Lifetime Nursing Home Use: Have Patterns of Use Changed?" *Medical Care*, 40 (2000): 965–975. A study conducted in the early 1990s, the results of which were widely quoted, showed that Americans had a 46 percent chance of requiring a nursing home before they died. This new study shows exactly the same probability.

Hospitals are under pressure to discharge patients as soon as possible. As a result, the average length of stay in a hospital for people over age 65 has plummeted from 12.6 days in 1970 to 5.8 days in 2001.

Public Health Service, "2001 National Hospital Discharge Survey," Advance Data No. 332 (Washington, D.C.: Government Printing Office, 2003). But older patients are no more ready to go home today than they were in 1970. Instead, they are discharged to a skilled nursing facility for "subacute" or "post-acute" care. Medicare pays for this kind of care but not for long-term stays.

2. American Association of Homes for the Aged, "Nursing Home Statistics," March 2001. The data are based on National Center for Health Statistics projections *(www.aahsa.org/public/backgrd/htm*, accessed September 2004).

3. K. G. Manton and X. Gu, "Changes in the Prevalence of Chronic Disability in the United States: Black and Non-Black Population Above Age 65 from 1982 to 1999," *Proceedings of the National Academy of Science*, 98 (2001): 6354–6359. As indicated by the title of the article, the rates cited are prevalence rates—the number of people with chronic disability per 1,000 people over the age of 65. They are not incidence rates, the number of new cases per 1,000 older individuals.

   The average number of impairments in activities of daily living (ADL) rises steadily as people move through the continuum of long-term care: home care, assisted living, and nursing home care. Recipients of ongoing services at home have a mean of 1.6 impairments, those in assisted living have a mean of 2.3, and those in nursing homes have a mean of 3.8. Quoted in Donald Redfoot and Sheel Pandya, *Before the Boom: Trends in Long-Term Supportive Services in Older Americans with Disabilities* (Washington, D.C.: AARP Public Policy Institute, 2002).

4. V. A. Freedman, L. G. Martin, and R. F. Schoen, "Recent Trends in Disability and Functioning Among Older Adults in the United States: A Systematic Review," *Journal of the American Medical Association*, 288 (2002): 3137–3146.

5. The MetLife Market Survey of Nursing Home and Home Health Care Costs, September 2004. *www.metlife.com*. For Boston, the average daily cost for a semiprivate room is $266, with a range of $185–$450.

6. A study conducted by the Centers for Medicare and Medicaid Services in 2003 found that 91 percent of nursing homes do not provide enough hours of care per resident per day to "avoid serious quality problems." Cited in M. J. Gibson, M. F. Friedman, and S. Gregory, "Beyond 50" (Washington, D.C.: AARP, 2003).

7. Erving Goffman, *Asylums: Essays on the Social Situation of Mental Patients and Other Inmates* (New York: Anchor Books, 1961).

8. The applicability of Goffman's model to the nursing home is elucidated by Charles Lidz, Lynn Fischer, and Robert Arnold in *The Erosion of Autonomy in Long-Term Care* (New York: Oxford University Press, 1992).

9. An eloquent article distinguishing between what most people want and what nursing homes strive for is Bart Collopy, "Safety and Independence: Rethinking Some Basic Concepts for Long-Term Care," in Laurence B. McCullough and Nancy L. Wilson, eds., *Long-Term Care Decisions: Ethical and Conceptual Dimensions* (Baltimore: Johns Hopkins University Press, 1995), pp. 137–152.

10. R. Kane, A. Caplan, E. Urv-Wong, et al., "Every Day Matters in the Lives of Nursing Home Residents: Wish for and Perception of Choice and Control," *Journal of the American Geriatrics Society,* 45 (1997): 1086–1093.

11. Marsha King, "The Pursuit of Happiness—Even in Old Age," *Seattle Times,* February 20, 1999.

12. S. Rimer, "Seattle's Elderly Finding a Home for Living, Not Dying," *New York Times,* November 22, 1998.

13. For a comprehensive description of the cultural change philosophy, see Wendy Lustbader, "The Pioneer Challenge: A Radical Change in the Culture of Nursing Homes," in L. Noelker and Z. Harel, eds., *Qualities of Care: Impact on Quality of Life* (New York: Springer, 2000), pp. 168–184. The mission and vision statements of the Pioneer movement are available on their Web site, *www.pioneermovement.org.*

14. George Engel put forward the biopsychosocial model of medicine in the late 1970s. Similar to holistic medicine, it centers on the interrelationship between mind and body and urges physicians to focus on the whole person.

15. Bill Thomas interviewed by Dale Bell on PBS, October 9, 2002, *www.pbs.org/thoushalthonor/eden/.*

16. Susan Dentzer, "A Nursing Home Alternative." Interview with Bill Thomas on "News Hour with Jim Lehrer," February 27, 2002, *www.pbs.org/newshour/bb/health/jan-june02/eden_2-27.html.*

17. The latest number of certified Eden facilities is available at *www.edenalternative.com,* and the latest statistics on Pioneer adherents are given at *www.pioneermovement.org.*

18. The Web site is *www.medicare.gov/nhcompare.*

19. Nursing homes are commonly given bucolic-sounding names, such as Happy Acres or Green Meadows. Because of its urban location, this nursing home does not have a pastoral name.

20. This makes sense for acute short-term facilities, dedicated to rehabilitation, and it is also a quality measure for these skilled nursing homes. It should be noted that the quality measures exempt patients who are dying from the requirement that function be maintained. However, facility staff systematically fail to record that a resident is terminally ill on the forms used to measure quality. See Steven Littlehale and Sam Simon, "Do Quality Measures Really Identify Quality of Care?" *Nursing Homes Long Term Care Management,* 54(5), May 2003.

21. It is unclear to me why infection rates are a measure of quality. Urinary tract infections and pneumonia are not contagious. A more appropriate indicator would focus on the extent to which the facility engaged in good preventive measures, such as vaccination against pneumococcal pneumonia and influenza.

22. The quality measures take into consideration whether the sore was acquired in the nursing home or elsewhere—to some extent. On the first "Minimum Data Set" form completed after Edna's return from the hospital, the pressure ulcer would not "count" against the facility. But if she still had it after 90 days—and deep ulcers often take that long to resolve—it would show up on the next MDS form.

23. A good, succinct summary of the bureaucratic structure of the regulatory system as well as the specific rules was put together by the American Medical Directors Association, "Synopsis of Federal Regulations in the Nursing Facility: Implications for Attending Physicians and Medical Directors," revised in January 2003 and posted on their Web site, *www.amda.com.*

24. One activist, Janet Tulloch, who was herself a nursing home resident, called the care plan "an instrument of terror" because of its role in a resident's daily life. Nursing homes now invite residents and their families to attend care planning meetings so the resident can in theory have a voice in shaping the process, but I have seen no studies looking at whether this is effective. See R. Kane, "Decision Making, Care Plans, and Life Plans," in McCullough and Wilson, eds., *Long-Term Care Decisions,* pp. 87–109.

25. The latest version of the MDS, version 2.0, is available on the CMS Web site at *www.cms.gov/medicaid/mds20*. It is made up of eighteen domains, ranging from mood to incontinence to visual function, and contains a total of 87 multiple-choice questions.

26. G. Winzelberg, "The Quest for Nursing Home Quality: Learning History's Lessons," *Archives of Internal Medicine*, 163 (2003): 2552–2556.

27. P. R. Katz, J. Karuza, J. Kolassa, and A. Hutsin, "Medical Practice with Nursing Home Residents: Results from the National Physician Professional Activities Census," *Journal of the American Geriatrics Society*, 45 (1997): 911–917. According to this report, 23 percent of general medical doctors and 15 percent of specialists provide care to nursing home patients.

28. Three articles in the *Journal of the American Geriatrics Society* reported on changes since the institution of the MDS. All were by the creators of the MDS, although the papers were introduced by a neutral authority and were accompanied by an independent editorial. See, for example, B. Fries, C. Hawes, J. Morris, et al., "Effect of the National Resident Assessment Instrument on Selected Health Conditions and Problems," *Journal of the American Geriatrics Society*, 45 (1997): 994–1001.

29. The Kaiser Family Foundation conducted a poll together with the Harvard School of Public Health in 1998, surveying 1,909 adult Americans on their knowledge and beliefs about Medicare. When asked "please tell me whether, to the best of your knowledge, the traditional Medicare program now pays for long term nursing home care," only 36 percent of the respondents knew the correct answer, although 44 percent of those over age 65 got the question right. Kaiser Family Foundation/Harvard School of Public Health National Survey on Medicare, October 20, 1998, *http://www.kff.org/medicare/1442-reform_pr.cfm*.

30. Mary A. Mendelson, *Tender Loving Greed* (New York: Knopf, 1974); Bruce C. Vladeck, *Unloving Care: The Nursing Home Tragedy* (New York: Basic Books, 1980).

31. R. Kane, "Long-Term Care and a Good Quality of Life: Bringing Them Closer Together," *The Gerontologist*, 41 (2003): 293–304.

32. In the first chapter of the Resident Assessment Instrument (RAI) manual, which describes how to use the MDS, the authors claim: "The RAI helps facility staff to look at residents holistically—as individuals for

whom quality of life and quality of care are mutually significant and necessary." It's hard to see evidence of this alleged focus on quality of life. See *www.cms.gov/medicaid/mds20.*

33. Bill Thomas interviewed by Dale Bell on PBS, October 9, 2002, *www .pbs.org/thoushalthonor/eden/.*

34. Report to Congress, "The Future Supply of Long-Term Care Workers in Relation to the Aging Baby Boom Generation," May 14, 2003, *http:// aspe.hhs.gov/daltcp/reports/ltcwork.htm,* accessed December 2004.

35. Robert Friedland, "Caregivers and Long-Term Care Needs in the 21st Century: Will Public Policy Meet the Challenge?" Georgetown University Long-Term Care Financing Project, Issue Brief, July 2004.

36. Nora Super, "Who Will Be There to Care? The Growing Gap between Caregiver Supply and Demand," National Health Policy Forum Background Paper, January 23, 2002, *http://www.nhpf.org/pdfs_bp/ BP_Caregivers_1-02.pdf.*

37. Ibid.

38. Robyn Stone, "Long-Term Care for the Elderly with Disabilities: Current Policy, Emerging Trends, and Implications for the Twenty-First Century," Milbank Memorial Fund, 2000, *www.milbank.org/reports/ 0008stone/.*

39. In 2001, nursing home facilities were the highest single Medicaid expenditure. Out of a $215 billion budget, Medicaid spent $53.1 billion on institutional long-term care. Centers for Medicare and Medicaid Services, "Program Information on Medicaid and State Children's Health Insurance Program (SCHIP)," 2004 Edition. *www.cms.hhs.gov/ charts/Medicaid/InfoMedicaid_schip.pdf.*

6. Assisted Living: Boon or Boondoggle?

1. As discussed in the previous chapter, the lifetime risk of entering a nursing home has remained unchanged since the early 1990s. B. C. Spillman and J. Lubitz, "New Estimates of Lifetime Nursing Home Use: Have Patterns of Use Changed?" *Medical Care,* 40 (2000): 965–973.

2. Web site of the Assisted Living Federation of America, *www.alfa.com.*

3. National Center for Assisted Living, *www.ncal.org/about/resident.htm.* Another 11 percent were discharged to a hospital.

4. CNN Interactive, "Assisted Living Gains Popularity Among Senior Citizens," August 13, 1998; *www.atriacom.com,* accessed October 20, 2003.

5. S. L. Stearns and L. A. Morgan, "Economics and Financing," in S. Zimmerman, P. Sloane, and J. Eckert, eds., *Assisted Living: Needs, Practices, and Policies in Residential Care for the Elderly* (Baltimore: Johns Hopkins University Press, 2001), pp. 271–291.

6. Andrew Goldstein, "Better Than a Nursing Home?" *Time* Magazine, August 13, 2001.

7. Donald Redfoot and Sheel Pandya, *Before the Boom: Trends in Long-Term Supportive Services for Older Americans with Disabilities* (Washington, D.C.: AARP Public Policy Institute, 2002), http://www.aarp.org/research/health/disabilities/aresearch-import-568-2002-15.html; Kelly Greene, "Assisted-Living Study Is Released," *Wall Street Journal,* April 30, 2003.

8. R. Kane, "Long-Term Care and a Good Quality of Life: Bringing Them Closer Together," *The Gerontologist,* 41 (2003): 293–304.

9. Not its real name. Like nursing homes, assisted living facilities usually have bucolic names, and some have suggested this indicates that older people are being put out to pasture in these "homes."

10. W. Andrew Achenbaum, *Old Age in the New Land* (Baltimore: Johns Hopkins University Press, 1978). Nearly two-thirds of the facilities in existence in the United States in 1939 were founded between 1875 and 1919. *23rd Annual Report of Charity of Massachusetts* (Boston: Wright and Potter Printing Company, 1900).

11. The story is told in somewhat greater detail in my article entitled "Long-Term Care Options for the Frail Elderly," *Journal of the American Geriatrics Society,* 37 (1989): 1198–1203.

12. Minutes of the Executive Board Meetings of the Ladies Unity Club, Inc., 1903–1923; also Admissions Records, Home for Aged Women. Archives, Schlesinger Library of Radcliff College, Cambridge, Massachusetts.

13. For a history of the development of old age homes, see M. Holstein and T. R. Cole, "Long-Term Care: A Historical Reflection," in Laurence B. McCullough and Nancy L. Wilson, eds., *Long-Term Care Decisions: Ethical and Conceptual Dimensions* (Baltimore: Johns Hopkins University Press, 1995), pp. 15–34.

14. Technology has the potential to be useful as well. Interactive computer

programs, for example, might be a means of reminding a person with dementia that it is mealtime. The computer could be infinitely patient and unfailingly polite in a way that human beings sometimes find difficult.

15. Goldstein, "Better Than a Nursing Home?"

16. P. D. Sloane, S. Zimmerman, and M. G. Ory, "Care for Persons with Dementia," in Zimmerman, Sloane, and Eckert, eds., *Assisted Living*, pp. 242–270.

17. V. Regnier and A. C. Scott, "Creating a Therapeutic Environment," in Zimmerman, Sloane, and Eckert, eds., *Assisted Living*, pp. 53–77.

18. This story of Ruth Cecil, age 79, was told by Kevin McCoy and Julie Appleby in one article of their series on assisted living: "Problems With Staffing, Training Can Cost Lives," *USA Today*, May 2004. The facility involved was The Fountains in Arizona.

19. The *USA Today* article cited in note 18 also describes the case of Grover McCurdy, an 85-year-old with dementia living in assisted living who died after choking on a chunk of meat. The facility was cited for failing to train its staff in first aid and cardiopulmonary resuscitation.

20. Catherine Hawes, a researcher in the long-term-care field, quotes a study from 2000 in which nine out of ten staff members at assisted living facilities thought that memory loss and confusion were normal with aging. Quoted by Kevin McCoy, "Poor Training Shows During Emergencies," *USA Today*, May 2004.

21. Another article in the *USA Today* series relates the story of Richard Maker at the Ridgecrest Retirement Center in Texaco. His doctor left three messages at the facility instructing them to stop Mr. Maker's Warfarin. The messages evidently were sent to a fax machine that was not checked. The patient continued to receive the same dose for the next few days and bled to death. See Kevin McCoy and Barbara Hansen, "Haven for Elderly May Expose Them to Deadly Risks," *USA Today*, May 2004.

22. U.S. Department of Health and Human Services, "A Profile of Older Americans, 2004," *http://www.aoa.gov/prof/Statistics/profile/2004/2004 profile.pdf*. In 2003, 9.9 percent of people over 65 had incomes under $15,000, while 50.4 percent had incomes over $35,000. Moreover, disability is correlated with poverty in the elderly, so that very poor peo-

ple (the government's definition of being at the poverty level) are twice as likely to report limitations in at least two activities of daily living (10.6 percent versus 5.2 percent).

23. J. Steinhauer, "As Assisted Living Centers Boom, Calls for Regulation Are Growing," *New York Times,* February 12, 2001.

24. General Accounting Office, "Assisted Living: Quality of Care and Consumer Protection in Four States," Washington, D.C., 1999 (GAO-HEHS-1399-27).

25. Andrew Goldstein, in his piece in *Time* Magazine, quotes Catherine Hawes from the University of North Carolina, Chapel Hill.

26. Barry Meier, "Experiment in Assisted Living Exposes Regulatory Confusion," *New York Times,* February 28, 2001.

27. L. Selhaus, "Economically Troubled Year for Assisted Living," *Provider Magazine,* August 2003.

28. The Assisted Living Workgroup, "Assessing Quality in Assisted Living: Guidelines for Federal and State Policy, State Regulation, and Operations. A Report to the U.S. Senate Special Committee on Aging," April 2003, *www.aahsa.org/alw.htm.*

29. Eric Carlson, "Policy Principles for Assisted Living," April 2003, *http://nsclc.org/articles/al_policyprinciples.htm,* p. 7.

30. Ibid.

31. Eric Carlson, "In the Sheep's Clothing of Resident Rights: Behind the Rhetoric of 'Negotiated Risk'" in Assisted Living," *National Association of Elder Law Attorneys Quarterly,* Spring 2003, pp. 4–9. Carlson argues that negotiated risk contracts are unenforceable and represent poor public policy. His point is that facilities cannot protect themselves from charges of *negligence,* if they are in fact negligent. He writes with biting sarcasm about the claims of assisted living facilities to be protecting the rights of residents to wear high heels or to eat cake. He also does not believe that nursing homes actually require residents to get up at designated times or dictate how they spend their days, indignantly citing the Nursing Home Reform Act, which requires that nursing homes provide care in a manner that "maintains or enhances each resident's dignity." Unfortunately, many nursing homes do require such things.

32. MetLife Mature Market Institute, "The MetLife Market Survey of Assisted Living Costs," October 2004, Westport, Connecticut, *www.Ma-*

ture MarketInstitute.com. MetLife conducted a telephone survey of assisted living facilities in all 50 states and the District of Columbia in July 2004. While the mean monthly cost was $2,524, there was tremendous geographic variability. The lowest base-rate average cost was $1,340 in Miami, and the highest was $4,327 in Stamford, Connecticut.

33. Stearns and Morgan, "Economics and Financing," in Zimmerman, Sloane, and Eckert, eds., *Assisted Living.*

34. Michael Nolin and Richard Mollica, "Residential Care/Assisted Living in the Changing Health Care Environment," in Zimmerman, Sloane, and Eckert, eds., *Assisted Living,* pp. 34–52.

35. M. J. Gibson, M. F. Friedman, S. Gregory, et al., "Beyond 50: A Report to the Nation on Independent Living and Disability" (Washington, D.C.: AARP, 2003). The authors report that people over 50 with disabilities strongly prefer independent living in their own homes. Above all, they want direct control over the "long-term supportive services" they receive. "Care" is held to be a paternalistic term. Given that what people want is a more caring attitude from their human helpers than is frequently the case, I think "care" rather than "services" is an eminently appropriate term.

36. NAELA Long-Term Care Task Force, "White Paper on Reforming the Delivery, Accessibility, and Financing of Long-Term Care in the United States," 2000, *www.naela.org/pdffiles/whitepaperltc1.pdf.* Medicare Part A covers hospital care; Medicare Part B covers laboratory tests and physicians' services; Medicare Part C is the name for "Medicare + Choice," the HMO alternative to conventional Medicare; Medicare Part D is the voluntary drug benefit, in effect as of 2006. The long-term-care benefit would be Medicare Part E.

37. Rosalie Kane and Keren Wilson, "Assisted Living at the Crossroads: Principles for Its Future," September 21, 2001, *http://www.ilru.org/html/training/webcasts/handouts/2002/10-09-JK/crossroads.html.* This excellent paper summarizes the history of assisted living, the principles that underlie it, and the challenges it faces as it tries to realize those principles. The authors conclude with twelve specific recommendations.

38. Ibid.

7. The Lure of Immortality

1. Andrew Pollack, "Forget Botox: Anti-Aging Pills May Be Next," *New York Times*, September 21, 2003.
2. The President's Council on Bioethics issued an impressive report on both the science and the ethics of life extension: *Beyond Therapy: Biotechnology and the Pursuit of Happiness* (Washington, D.C., 2003). The report, which includes an entire chapter on "Ageless Bodies," is available on the Internet at *www.bioethics.gov/reports/beyondtherapy/chapter4.html*.
3. In a report of the experience of 119 patients with the ICD, most describe the shocks as "severe." Common descriptions include "a blow to the body" and "a spasm causing the body to jump." Fully 23 percent said they dread the shocks; 5 percent said they would prefer to be without the ICD and take their chances. Patients in other studies have reported increased anxiety, depression, and a diminished quality of life. See M. Ahmad, L. Bloomstein, M. Roelke, et al., "Patients' Attitudes Toward Implanted Defibrillator Shocks," *Pacing and Clinical Electrophysiology*, 23 (2000): 934–938.
4. Despite the widespread precedent for discontinuing unwanted, burdensome treatment, many cardiologists express dismay at the prospect of turning off defibrillators. Some refuse to do so. See Paul Mueller, C. Christopher Hook, and David Hayes, "Ethical Analysis of Withdrawal of Pacemaker or Implantable Cardioverter-Defibrillator Support at the End of Life," *Mayo Clinic Proceedings*, 78 (2003): 959–963.
5. Jonathan Swift, *Gulliver's Travels* (New York: Grolier, 1976), pp. 246–248.
6. As the medical specialty of geriatrics emerged into adulthood, a full-blown controversy developed between those who thought geriatrics was leading to a compression of morbidity and those who thought it should but it wasn't. The seminal article was by J. Fries, "Aging, Natural Death, and the Compression of Mortality," *New England Journal of Medicine*, 303 (1980): 130–135.
7. Richard Miller, "Extending Life: Scientific Prospects and Political Obstacles," *Milbank Quarterly*, 80 (2002): 155–174.

8. Leonard Guarente and Cynthia Kenyon, "Genetic Pathways That Regulate Ageing in Model Organisms," *Nature,* 408 (2000): 255–262.

9. Vernon Ingram, "The Sickle Cell Story," *www.bioinfo.org.cn/book/great %20Experiments/great2.htm,* accessed April 28, 2004.

10. An excellent book about the scientific pursuit of life extension, which features an engaging and extensive account of the activities and antics of Michael West, is Stephen Hall's *Merchants of Immortality: Chasing the Dream of Human Life Extension* (Boston: Houghton Mifflin, 2003).

11. Michael West relates the story of his mother's death and indicates that he stood by her hospital bed, "hating death." See Michael West, "Back to Immortality: The Opportunities and Challenges of Therapeutic Cloning," *Life Extension Magazine,* November 2003.

12. Reports of an "obesity epidemic" in the United States have been multiplying. One study found that 30 percent of Americans are obese, leading to an estimated $75 billion per year in medical costs. Marian Uhlman, "Obesity Cost to US $75.1 Billion, Study Says," *Philadelphia Inquirer,* January 22, 2004.

13. Mark Lane, Donald Ingram, and George Roth, "The Serious Search for an Anti-Aging Pill," *Scientific American,* August 2002.

14. The U.S. Census Bureau figures give the number of American centenarians as 88,289 in 2004, up from 50,454 in 2003 and 37,306 in 1990. Quoted in the MetLife "Demographic Profile: Americans 65+", *http:// www.metlife.com/WPSAssets/78466792201110468360V1F65+Profile-10-10-04.pdf.*

15. The information about centenarians is from the Web site for the New England Centenarian Study, *www.bumc.bu.edu/centenarian.* John Rowe and Robert Kahn coined the phrase "successful aging" to indicate that people do have some control over whether they remain robust into old age. They based their conclusions on an eight-year study of over 1,000 well-functioning older people known as the MacArthur Foundation Study. Their book is entitled *Successful Aging* (New York: Pantheon Books, 1998).

16. *Houston Chronicle* News Service, "Believed to be World's Oldest,

Woman in France Dies at 122," August 4, 1997, p. 1 *(www.chron.con/ content/chronicle/page1/97/08/05/calment.html)*.

17. The Okinawans were brought to public attention by Bradley Willcox, Craig Willcox, and Makoto Suzaki in their book *The Okinawa Program: How the World's Longest-Lived People Achieve Everlasting Health —And How You Can Too* (New York: Clarkson Potter, 2001).

18. Gina Kolata, "Patients in Florida Lining Up for All That Medicare Covers," *New York Times,* September 13, 2003.

19. Studies have found a strong association between higher spending and greater intensity of end-of-life care and a lack of association between higher spending and increased discretionary surgery or effective care. During the last six months of life, the additional spending in Miami (as compared to Portland and Minneapolis) purchased 6.55 times more visits to medical specialists, 2.16 times more ICU admissions, and 2.13 times more hospital days. Rates of effective care (interventions of proven value such as vaccination against pneumonia) were lower in Miami than in Minneapolis. See John Wennberg, Megan Cooper, and Susan Tolle, "Variability in End-of-Life Care in the United States," in R. Morrison, Diane Meier, and Carol Capello, eds., *Geriatric Palliative Care* (New York: Oxford University Press, 2003), pp. 3–16.

20. Oliver Wendell Homes, noted turn of the (twentieth) century physician, wrote the poem "The Deacon's Masterpiece" or "The Wonderful One-Hoss Shay." It begins:

> Have you heard of the wonderful one-hoss shay,
> That was built in such a logical way
> It ran a hundred years to a day,
> And then, of a sudden, it—ah, but stay,
> I'll tell you what happened without delay,
> Scaring the parson into fits,
> Frightening people out of their wits,—
> Have you ever heard of that, I say?

The poem's concluding verse is:

What do you think the parson found,
When he got up and stared around?
The poor old chaise in a heap or mound,
As if it had been to the mill and ground!
You see, of course, if you're not a dunce,
How it went to pieces all at once,—
All at once, and nothing first,
Just as bubbles do when they burst.

Quoted from *www.readbookonline.net/readOnLine/1157.*

21. K. A. Hesse, "Terminal Care of the Very Old: Changes in the Way We Die," *Archives of Internal Medicine,* 155 (1995): 1513–1518.

22. S. R. Cummings and L. J. Milton, "Epidemiology and Outcomes of Osteoporotic Fractures," *Lancet,* 359 (2002): 1761–1767. The lifetime risk of breaking a hip for women from age 50 is 17 percent, while for men it is 6 percent. But it is important to realize that 30 percent of all osteoporotic fractures occur in men. As the risk rises with age in women, it does likewise in men.

23. W. Mondale, K. Pohl, and P. Hewitt, *Meeting the Challenge of Global Aging* (Washington, D.C.: CSIS Press, 2002).

24. The projections for the old age dependency ratio vary. The Social Security Administration tries to predict its financing needs for the coming 75 years. It typically makes both a worst-case scenario prediction and a best-case scenario. Its worst-case prediction is 56/100 in 2075. However, a new study by two demographers at the University of California at Berkeley suggests that there is a 25 percent probability that the ratio will be higher than that, and a 2.5 percent chance that it might even reach 82/100. "Social Security: The Long View. Making the Case for Pessimism," *Business Week Online:* Economic Trends, January 14, 2002, *www.businessweek.com:/print/magazine/content/02_02/c3765072.htm?mz.*

25. I am using Richard Miller's estimate of a mean age at death of 112 years, which is in turn based on the assumption that mean lifespan could be increased 40 percent, the rate of improvement achieved in rodents. See Miller, "Extending Life." Miller's estimates were chosen be-

cause he strikes me as one of the most scientifically credible of the believers in the possibility of extending longevity.

26. The data on life expectancy are from the U.S. Census Bureau, International Data Base, Summary of Demographics, *www.census.gov*. This site allows you to click on any country in the world and find out not only the life expectancy at birth, fertility rate, current population, and projections for the future, but also to look at a depiction of the age pyramid, which gives a graphic representation of the shape of the population.

27. For a comprehensive philosophical analysis of longevity and immortality, see Christine Overall's *Aging, Death, and Human Longevity: A Philosophical Inquiry* (Berkeley: University of California Press, 2003). The book is a totally humorless discussion of completely implausible states, but for those with a taste for this kind of analysis, it does address at length questions such as whether it would be good to live forever and whether death is evil. The "apologist" perspective is presented, rather more eloquently, by Daniel Callahan in his book *What Price Better Health? Hazards of the Research Imperative* (Berkeley: University of California Press, 2003).

28. The President's Council on Bioethics, *Beyond Therapy: Biotechnology and the Pursuit of Happiness*, chapter 4, "Ageless Bodies," *www.bio ethics.gov/report/beyondtherapy/chapter4.html.*, p. 21.

29. Centers for Disease Control, Morbidity and Mortality Weekly Report, "Achievements in Public Health, 1900–1997," July 30, 1999, vol. 48, pp. 621–629. Much of the 29-year increase in life expectancy at birth is due to the fall in infant and childhood mortality. The leading causes of death in 1900 were pneumonia, tuberculosis, and diarrheal disease. A full 40 percent of the deaths due to these three conditions occurred in children under 5 years of age.

30. Peter Laslett, a demographer, makes a number of fascinating arguments about the effects of changes in age distribution in a population in the chapter "Necessary Knowledge: Age and Ageing in the Societies of the Past," in David Kertzer and Peter Laslett, eds., *Aging in the Past: Demography, Society, and Old Age* (Berkeley: University of California Press, 1995), pp. 3–77. He says that life expectancy at age 15 is a far

better measure than life expectancy at birth to capture the characteristic pattern of aging in a society.

31. For a discussion of the shift from veneration to vilification, see David Hackett Fischer, *Growing Old in America* (New York: Oxford University Press, 1978).

32. Ibid. Fischer provides fascinating examples of the ways in which the early American veneration for the elderly was manifested. He writes, "In the seventeenth century, and still more in the eighteenth, a single style appeared for all age groups, designed to flatter the old. Hair was hidden beneath a wig, or powdered and made white as if by old age" (*Growing Old in America,* p. 86). Similarly, the cut of men's clothes was intended to make even young people look old: the backs of coats were designed to "make the spine appear to be bent by the weight of many years" (p. 87).

33. Jewish Publication Society of America, *The Writings (Kethubim)* (Philadelphia, 1982).

34. For an excellent summary of past quests for immortality, as well as a good description of what is biologically feasible, see S. Jay Olshansky and Bruce A. Carnes, *The Quest for Immortality: Science at the Frontiers of Aging* (New York: Norton, 2001).

35. Ernest Becker, *The Denial of Death* (New York: The Free Press, 1973). Becker argues that the unique human awareness of our mortality creates a sense of anxiety in people, and the denial of death is thus a basic psychological protective trait. Suppression of our awareness of our mortality is critical for us to be able to function from day to day. Immortality projects—which can be very productive or can be extremely destructive—are our way to feel permanent and invulnerable.

36. Leon Kass, *Life, Liberty, and the Defense of Dignity: The Challenge for Bioethics* (San Francisco: Encounter Books, 2002). Kass gives four reasons for favoring finitude. The first is what he calls interest and engagement: he argues that if the human lifespan were increased, even by a mere twenty years, the pleasures of life would not increase proportionately. Then he discusses seriousness and aspiration, the importance of mortality as a spur to meaningful activity. He also says that beauty and love exist only by contrast with decay and death. Finally, he writes of virtue and moral excellence: "Through moral courage, en-

durance, greatness of soul, generosity, devotion to justice—in acts great and small—we rise above our mere creatureliness, spending the precious coinage of the time of our lives for the sake of the noble and the holy" (p. 268).

8. Making the Most of the Retirement Years

1. The story of the group of children is told by David Gumpert in a memoir based on the diaries of his aunt, Inge Bleier: *Inge: A Girl's Journey Through Nazi Europe* (Grand Rapids: William Eerdmans, 2004).

2. This was the finding of the MacArthur Report on Successful Aging, as quoted by Rebecca Gardyn, "Retirement Redefined," *American Demographics*, November 2002, p. 52.

3. Susan Dominus, "Life in the Age of Old, Old Age," *New York Times Magazine*, February 22, 2004, p. 26.

4. *www.npr.org/about/people/bios/dschorr.html*, accessed April 15, 2004. See also Daniel Schorr's memoir, *Staying Tuned: A Life in Journalism* (New York: Pocket Books, 2001).

5. Betty Friedan, *The Fountain of Age* (New York: Simon and Schuster, 1993).

6. San Diego Museum of Art, "Grandma Moses in the 21st Century," *http://www.absolutearts.com/artsnews/2001/07/01/28787.html*.

7. Gardyn, "Retirement Redefined."

8. Erikson first articulated the stages of development in his seminal work, *Childhood and Society* (New York: Norton, 1950). An interesting article that expands on Erikson's seventh stage (the eighth stage is "integrity vs. despair") is Charles Slater, "Generativity Versus Stagnation: An Elaboration of Erikson's Adult Stage of Human Development," *Journal of Adult Development*, 10 (2003): 53–65.

9. This account is from Marc Freedman, *Prime Time* (New York: Public Affairs, 1999), pp. 87–88.

10. Marc Freedman, founder and CEO of Civic Ventures, has proposed passage of a federal Third Age Bill—the third age being the term for the post-retirement years. Analogous to the GI Bill which helped returning U.S. soldiers after World War II reintegrate into society, it

would create a national service corps of people over 55, subsidizing new programs and providing a stipend and health benefits to participants. The political will to support such a bill has been absent, but the Experience Corps is a modest version that grew up in the private sector.

11. Freedman, *Prime Time,* pp. 183–216.

12. See the Civic Ventures Web site, *www.civicventures.org.*

13. In the 1960s, families first began advocating for a broader federal role in providing what would become known as FAPE, free appropriate public education, for children with assorted disabilities. In 1970, Congress passed the Education of the Handicapped Act (PL 91-230). This was updated in 1997 to IDEA, the Individuals with Disabilities Education Act.

14. Steve Gillon traces the development of the new urbanism in his descriptions of Elizabeth Platter-Zyberk and Andres Duaney, two of the prototypical baby boomers whose life stories he tells in *Boomer Nation: The Largest and Richest Generation Ever, and How It Changed America* (New York: Free Press, 2004).

15. The course catalog is available online at *http://www.unca.edu/ncccr/Catalog/FALL05/.*

16. The importance of social capital, its decline in America since World War II, and prospects for creating new forms of social capital are discussed in the influential book *Bowling Alone: The Collapse and Revival of American Community* by Robert Putnam (New York: Simon and Schuster, 2000). Social capital was first described by a Progressive reformer in 1916 as "those tangible substances [that] count for most in the daily lives of people: namely good will, fellowship, sympathy, and social intercourse among the individuals and families who make up a social unit . . . The community as a whole will benefit by the cooperation of all its parts, while the individual will find in his associations the advantages of the help, the sympathy, and the fellowship of his neighbors" (p. 19); Putnam is quoting Lydia Judson Hanifan, "The Rural School Community Center," *Annals of the American Academy of Political and Social Science,* 67 (1916): 130–138.

17. In business and industry, mentoring has been found to be helpful in attracting, retaining, and promoting junior employees. It has im-

proved both individual and corporate performance. In higher education, mentoring can help junior faculty advance. See G. Luna and D. Cullen, "Empowering the Faculty. Mentoring: Redirected and Renewed," *www.ntf.com/html/lib/bib/95–3dg.htm*, accessed April 27, 2004.

18. Willard Gaylin and Bruce Jennings, *The Perversion of Autonomy: The Proper Uses of Coercion and Constraints in a Liberal Society* (New York: The Free Press, 1996).

19. Daniel Yankelovich, *New Rules: Seeking Self-Fulfillment in a World Turned Upside Down* (New York: Random House, 1981); Alan Wolfe, *One Nation, After All: What Middle-Class Americans Really Think about God, Country, Family, Racism, Welfare, Immigration, Homosexuality, Work, The Right, The Left, and Each Other* (New York: Penguin Books, 1999); Putnam, *Bowling Alone*.

20. Gaylin and Jennings, *The Perversion of Autonomy*, pp. 58, 73.

21. A fascinating book summarizing the many studies about just how much choice patients really want is Carl Schneider's *The Practice of Autonomy: Patients, Doctors, and Medical Decisions* (New York: Oxford University Press, 1998). He concludes that the vast majority of patients want to be informed about their illness. They want a diagnosis. They want to understand the prognosis. They even want to know the options. But they want their physician to recommend, perhaps to select, a course of treatment.

22. Ingelfinger expressed his views in an address at Harvard Medical School, the George W. Gay Lecture, in 1977. His remarks were reprinted in an essay called "Arrogance" in the *New England Journal of Medicine*, 303 (1980): 1507.

Finale

1. MetLife Mature Market Institute, "A Profile of American Baby Boomers: Demographic Profile" (based on U.S. Census Bureau statistics, 2000).

2. We have direct evidence that exercise can improve function in older people: see, for example, M. Nelson, J. Layne, M. Bornstein, et al., "The Effect of Multidimensional Home-Based Exercise on Functional Per-

formance in Elderly People," *Journals of Gerontology Series A: Biological Medical Science,* 59 (2004): 154–160. We also have evidence that lower-extremity weakness, which can presumably be improved with exercise, predicts future disability. See J. Guralnick, L. Ferrucci, E. Simonsick, et al., "Lower-Extremity Function in Persons Over the Age of 70 Years as a Predictor of Subsequent Disability," *New England Journal of Medicine,* 332 (1995): 556–561.

3. F. Mookadam and H. Arthur, "Social Support and Its Relationship to Morbidity and Mortality After Acute Myocardial Infarction: Systematic Overview," *Archives of Internal Medicine,* 164 (2004): 1514–1518; S. Cummings, S. Phillips, M. Wheat, et al., "Recovery of Function After Hip Fracture: The Role of Social Supports," *Journal of the American Geriatrics Society,* 36 (1988): 801–806; S. Bassuk, T. Glass, and L. Berkman, "Social Disengagement and Incident Cognitive Decline in Community-Dwelling Older Persons," *Annals of Internal Medicine,* 131 (1999): 165–173.

4. George Agich discusses the philosophical underpinnings of the concept of autonomy as it relates to individuals with physical and/or cognitive impairment in *Autonomy and Long-Term Care* (New York: Oxford University Press, 1993). Agich does not reject autonomy as irrelevant or unimportant to frail elders; rather, he seeks to create a framework that "shift[s] . . . attention from autonomy as independence to actual autonomy as it appears in the everyday world of life" (p. 12).

5. I argued earlier in the book that no single life-style modification results in profound changes in risk. Nonetheless, for an individual who develops a condition that he might otherwise have avoided, the repercussions are substantial. Moreover, while the effect of any given intervention is small, the cumulative effect of multiple behavioral changes may be large.

6. Susan Diem, John Lantos, and James Tulsky, "Cardiopulmonary Resuscitation on Television—Miracles and Misinformation," *New England Journal of Medicine,* 334 (1996): 1578–1582.

7. D. Murphy, A. Murray, B. Robinson, and E. Campion, "Outcomes of Cardiopulmonary Resuscitation in the Elderly," *Annals of Internal Medicine,* 111 (1989): 199–205. These data are a bit old. It is possible

that the automated external defibrillator, now increasingly available in public places such as airports and shopping malls, will modify the statistics. But the fundamental reality is that CPR works best for people with an isolated electrical problem of the heart, not for individuals with assorted other medical problems, in whom cardiac arrest is simply the final common pathway to death.

8. M. Brodie, U. Foehr, C. Rideout, et al., "Community Health Information Through the Entertainment Media," *Health Affairs*, 20 (2001): 192–199.

9. Joseph Turow and Rachel Gans, "As Seen on TV: Health Policy Issues in TV's Medical Dramas. A Report to the Kaiser Family Foundation," July 2002, *www.kff.org.*

10. Mollyann Brodie, Drew Altman, LeeAnn Brady, and Lindsay Heberling, "A Study of Media Coverage of Health Policy, 1997–2000," *Columbia Journalism Review Supplement*, January/February 2002.

11. Maria Vesperi, "Forty-Nine Plus: Shifting Images of Aging in the Media," in *Reinventing Aging: Baby Boomers and Civic Engagement* (Boston: Center for Health Communication, Harvard School of Public Health, 2004).

12. Several recent movies have contributed to the public understanding of aging: *Iris* in 2001 (based on John Bayley's *Elegy for Iris;* New York: St. Martin's Press, 1999); *Innocence* in 2000; and *The Barbarian Invasions* in 2003. They followed the earlier popular movies *A Woman's Tale* (1991), *Driving Miss Daisy* (1989), *Trip to Bountiful* (1985), and *On Golden Pond* (1981), some of the first of the genre. The last few years have also seen a spate of novels and memoirs dealing with the care of an aging parent, often a parent with Alzheimer's disease. See Sue Miller, *The Story of My Father: A Memoir* (New York: Knopf, 2003); Judy Levine, *Do You Remember Me? A Father, a Daughter, and a Season for the Self* (New York: Free Press, 2004); and Michael Stein, *This Room Is Yours* (Sag Harbor, N.Y.: Permanent Press, 2004.)

13. This and the following paragraphs draw extensively on Thomas Cole, *The Journey of Life: A Cultural History of Aging in America* (New York: Cambridge University Press, 1992). The quotation in this paragraph is from p. 231.

14. Ibid., p. 239.

15. George Vaillant, *Aging Well: Surprising Guideposts to a Happier Life from the Landmark Harvard Study of Adult Development* (Boston: Little, Brown, 2002), pp. 309–310. Vaillant's study is based on three groups: a sample of 268 Harvard graduates born about 1920 (by definition, all male); a sample of 456 socially disadvantaged men from the inner city born about 1930; and a sample of 90 middle-class, intellectually gifted women born about 1910.

Acknowledgments

MY GREATEST debt in writing this book is to my patients. Their struggles and predicaments, their triumphs and misfortunes form the basis of the stories I relate. The difficulties my patients encounter—in prodding health care institutions to respond to their needs, in locating suitable nursing homes or assisted living facilities, and in finding meaning in life despite old age and disability—have stimulated me to think and read and ultimately to write about what's right and what's wrong with geriatric care today.

I am also grateful for the insightful comments offered by my academic colleagues at the Department of Ambulatory Care and Prevention of Harvard Medical School/Harvard Pilgrim Health Care: Jim Sabin, Steve Pearson, and Mary Barton each read and critiqued assorted chapters of the manuscript. I thank my clinical colleagues at Harvard Vanguard Medical Associates who drew on their wisdom, derived from extensive experience caring for older patients and their families, in giving feedback on yet other chapters: Bob Buxbaum, Gisela Perkins, and Mark Yurkofsky. Most importantly, I thank my editors at Harvard University Press: Elizabeth Knoll believed from our first meeting that I had a perspective on aging that deserved attention and sensed my passion for improving the way we think about and care for older people. Through the various revisions of the book, she gently insisted that I not bury this passion under a mountain of statistics nor coat it with a veneer of academic policy lingo. She encouraged me to speak from the heart and to consign the more statistical and technical parts of my argument to the endnotes. Mary Ellen Geer made the kinds of nuanced, insightful, and sensible stylistic suggestions that every author hopes for.

A resounding thank-you goes to one of the outside readers for Harvard University Press, whose trenchant critique helped shape the final version of the book. And the greatest thanks of all goes to my husband, Larry, who never tires of reminding me that I'm happiest when I'm working on a book.

Index

AARP: The Magazine, 5, 274
Acetaminophen, 20, 64–65, 127, 201
Acute illnesses, and Medicare, 94, 102, 113, 119
Adult day care, 113–114, 192
Advertisements, 266
African Americans, 12
AgeLab, 275
Agency for Healthcare Research and Quality, 274
Aging process, 195–196, 205–214, 218–224, 267–268, 284–285
AIDS, 6, 101, 118
Almshouses, 166
Alterra Corporation, 169, 178–180, 188
Alzheimer's disease, 5–7, 45, 63, 65, 72, 77, 84–85, 104, 107, 124, 168, 205
American Association of Homes and Services for the Aging, 283
American Association of Retired Persons, 5, 225–226, 273–274
American Cancer Society, 81
American College of Physicians, 16
American Health Care Association, 283
American Heart Association, 81

American Medical Association, 15–16, 71–72
Americans for Better Care of the Dying, 278–279
Americans with Disabilities Act, 243
Anemia, 118, 198, 207–208, 238
Angola, 220
Annals of Internal Medicine, 18, 22
Annual checkups, 15–19, 23, 26, 32, 36
Antibiotics, 41–43, 64–65, 69, 74
Anticoagulant drugs, 58–59
Antidepressant drugs, 34–35
Antihypertensive drugs, 30–31
Anti-inflammatory drugs, 20
Antioxidants, 210
Anxiety, 35, 127
Arrhythmia, 50, 55, 58, 199–200, 238
Arthritis, 7, 19–21, 34, 56, 106, 124, 197–198
Arthroscopy, 20–21
Asheville, N. C., 246
Aspirin, 80
Assisted living, 9–10, 124, 157, 161–164, 170–178, 255, 283; growing need for facilities, 151–153; number of units,

Assisted living *(continued)*
159–160; caregivers in, 163, 182–183;
and old age homes, 164–167; and
Medicare/Medicaid, 167, 178, 182,
188–191, 193; benefits/drawbacks of,
167–168, 190–191; and dementia,
168–170, 190; costs, 178, 191; regulation of, 178–182; quality of care/life,
181–183, 192; proposed levels of care,
184–185, 191–192; negotiated risk
contracts, 185–188; as communities,
262–263
Assisted Living Federation of America,
159
Atherosclerosis, 30
Atlantic Monthly, 244
Australia, 57
Autonomy, 10, 170, 181, 184–185, 250–
253, 259

Baby boomers, population statistics,
123, 257
Balanced Budget Act, 157
Baptist Home, 165
Becker, Ernest, 223
Belgium, 227–228
Beta-blockers, 80
Biopsies, 33
Birth control, 221
Birthrate, 218
Blood clots, 22, 58–59, 96–97
Blood disorders: anemia, 118, 198, 207–
208, 238; sickle cell disease, 118, 207–
208; leukemia, 119; multiple
myeloma, 238
Blood pressure, 16–17, 30–31, 56
Blood tests, 39–40
Blood-thinning drugs, 58–59, 96–98
Board and care facilities, 167
Body scans, 27–29
Bone disorders: osteoarthritis, 7, 19–21,

197–198; osteoporosis, 22, 35, 111,
121, 215–216; hip fractures, 22, 34–
36, 56, 141–142, 198, 215, 258
Bone marrow transplants, 119
Bone mass, 22, 35
Boston, Mass., 16, 28, 165, 188, 247
Botox injections, 3–4, 14, 219
Brain tumors, 85–88
Breast cancer, 11, 17, 22–23, 27, 30, 32,
61, 120
Breaux, John, 180
Britain, 89–90
Burnap Free Home for Aged Women, 165
Bush, George W., 154, 224
Bypass surgery, 12, 47–48, 51–52

Caenorhabditis elegans, 206–207, 209
Caffeine, 21
Calcium, 216
California, 28, 79, 179
Calment, Jeanne, 212
Caloric restriction, 209–210
Cambridge, Mass., 165
Canada, 15–16, 81
Cancer, 69, 75, 89, 115–116; breast, 11,
17, 22–23, 27, 30, 32, 61, 120; pros-
tate, 12–17, 24–27, 29, 33–34; colon,
17, 30; uterine, 22; cervical, 31, 259;
larynx, 43–44; skin, 196–197; multi-
ple myeloma, 238
Cardiac stents, 48, 257
Cardiomyopathy, 240, 243
Cardiopulmonary resuscitation (CPR),
70, 76, 78–79, 202, 257, 264
Caregivers, 8, 262; in hospices, 90; in
nursing homes, 127–134, 145, 147,
151–155; in assisted living, 163, 182–
184
Cash and Counseling, 276
Cataract surgery, 198
Catholicism/Catholics, 66–67, 77

CBS, 233
Centenarians, 211–214, 218, 284
Center for Creative Retirement, 246–247
Centers for Medicare and Medicaid Services, 149–150, 156
Cervical cancer, 31, 259
Chanina, Rabbi, 68
Checkups. *See* Annual checkups
Child mortality, 221
Chinese Americans, 112
Cholecystectomy, 42, 47–48
Cholecystitis, 42–43
Cholesterol, 21, 31, 56, 184, 257–258
Chronic illnesses, and Medicare, 94, 102, 112–114, 119, 263
Civic Ventures, 236–237, 286
Clare Bridge, 169, 188
Clinton, Bill, 154
CNN, 160, 234
Codeine, 201
Cole, Thomas, 267–268
Collective for Medical Decisions, 77–79
College courses, 229–230, 245–247
College for Seniors, 246
Colon cancer, 17, 30
Colonoscopy, 13, 30
Colorado, 77–79
Comfort, promotion of, 64–66, 72, 81, 88–91, 103, 115
Comprehensive care, 107–108, 111–114, 116–118
Computerized axial tomography (CAT) scans, 28
Concentration camps, 228–229
Confusion, 45, 99
Congestive heart failure, 56–58, 238
Congress, U.S., 3, 180, 243. *See also specific acts*
Consumer Consortium on Assisted Living, 180–181
Co-payments, 116–117

CPK-MB blood test, 39–40
Craigslist, 249
Creative arts therapy, 147
Cystic fibrosis, 207–208

Day health care centers, 113–114, 192
Death, 6, 63; ethical issues, 66–83; physician-assisted suicide, 83, 88, 91, 252–253; and hospice care, 87–91; as part of life cycle, 209, 220–222
Death rates, hospital, 46
Deductibles, 116–117
Deep vein thrombosis, 22, 96–98
Defibrillators, 199–203
Dehydration, 65, 75, 143–144
Delirium, 41
Dementia, 7–8, 22, 36, 44, 72, 74–75, 78, 99, 107, 118, 121, 153, 161–163, 168–170, 178, 183, 190, 192, 199–202, 205, 258. *See also* Alzheimer's disease
Dentistry, 113
Dentures, 111, 114
Denver, Col., 16, 77–79
Depression, 25–26, 35, 99, 238
Dermatology, 196–197
Diabetes, 17, 184, 187
Diarrhea, 26
Diet, 3, 6–7, 67, 184, 187, 209–210, 213, 255, 258, 267
Disease management, 57–61
DNA, 208
Down syndrome, 241, 244
Drugs. *See* Prescription drugs
Duaney, Andres, 244

Eagan, Minn., 168–169, 188
Ecclesiastes, 222
Echocardiograms, 49
Eden Alternative, 134–136, 151, 282
Education, health, 260–261, 264–266
Education of the Handicapped Act, 243

Elderhostel, 225, 247
Electrocardiograms (EKGs), 39–40, 50
Elixir, 195, 206–207
Emphysema, 56, 114
Employment, and health insurance, 118–119
End-of-life care, 88–91, 94, 102–103, 110–111, 114–120, 253, 277–279
Erikson, Erik, 235
Estrogen, 21–23
Evercare, 60
Evergreen, 170
Evidence-based medicine, 18–19, 23, 29, 81
Exercise, 3, 6–7, 35, 209, 255, 257–258, 261–262, 267
Experience Corps, 236–237, 286
Extending life. *See* Life, prolongation of
Eye disorders: macular degeneration, 7, 56; glaucoma, 111; laser surgery, 120–121; cataract surgery, 198
Eyeglasses, 93, 111, 114

Facelifts, 4
Faith communities, 244, 247–248
Faith in Action, 276
Falls, 34–36, 141, 186, 259. *See also* Hip fractures
Family Caregiver Alliance, 277
Feeding tubes, 109–110
Fixx, Jim, 3
Florida, 79, 213–214, 223, 244–245
Flu shots, 111, 216
Fortune, 160
Foster Grandparents, 236, 286
Fountain of Youth legend, 223
Frailty, 7–8, 36–37, 40–43, 45–47, 56, 94, 101, 106–114, 118–121, 131, 135, 205, 237–238
France, 228–229
Free radicals, 210

Fried, Linda, 237
Friedan, Betty: *The Fountain of Age,* 5, 234
Fuss Center for Research on Aging and Intergenerational Studies, 247
Futility, 69–72, 76–83

Gallbladder attack, 42–43, 47–48
Gardening, 269
Gaylin, Willard, 251
General Accounting Office, 180
Generativity, 235, 269
Gene therapy, 206–210, 267
Geriatrics, 9, 41–42, 120, 205
German Ladies Aid Society, 165
Germany, 218, 227
Geron, 208–209
Glaucoma, 111
Glioblastoma, 85–88
Gray Panthers, 181
Green House, 135–136
Growth hormones, 219
Growth House, 277

Hair coloring, 3, 14
Health care proxies, 65–66, 70–72, 76–77, 242
Health education, 260–261, 264–266
Health insurance, 12, 118–119
Health maintenance organizations, 60, 116–117, 260
Healthy People, 11
Hearing aids, 93, 111, 114
Heart attack, 3, 22, 30–31, 36, 38–40, 45, 48, 55–57, 80, 199, 257–258
Heart-bypass surgery, 12, 47–48, 51–52
Heart disease. *See* Congestive heart failure; Heart attack
Heart failure, 56–58, 238
Heart pumps, 114, 120
Heart stents, 48, 257

Hennepin County Hospital, 70–71
Henry J. Kaiser Family Foundation, 280
Heparin, 96–98
High blood pressure, 30–31, 56
Hill-Burton Act, 167
Hip fractures, 22, 34–36, 56, 141–142, 198, 215, 258–259
Holmes, Oliver Wendell, 214
Home care, 57–58, 60, 87, 94–103, 107–108, 113, 115, 124, 151–154, 157, 262
Home health aides, 55, 105–106, 154
Hospices, 42, 87–91, 102–103, 110–111, 114–116, 277–278
Hospital-acquired infections, 46
Hospitalization, 52, 66, 72, 123, 148, 200–201, 217–218; adverse effects of, 40–47; and disease management, 58–60; and Medicare/Medicaid, 94, 96–103, 109–110, 113, 115, 120
Houston, Texas, 78–79
Hysterectomy, 22

Immortality, 6–7, 10, 203–205, 211, 223–224
Impotence, 25–26, 29
Incontinence, 24–26, 29, 121, 131–132, 168, 183
Individualism, 250, 267. *See also* Autonomy
Infection rates, 46, 141
Influenza vaccinations, 111, 216
Ingelfinger, Franz, 252
Intensive care, 111, 116–118
Intensive care units, 66, 70–72, 78, 82, 113
Intergenerational campus communities, 245–248, 263
Intermediate care, 42–47, 60–61, 94
International Longevity Center–USA, 284
Internet, 248–250

Ischemia, 50
Italy, 155, 218

Japan, 155, 212–213, 220
Jennings, Bruce, 251
Johns Hopkins University, 237, 276
Johnson Foundation, 112, 276
Judah the Prince, Rabbi, 67
Judaism/Jews, 67–68, 227–229

Kaiser Foundation, 280
Kass, Leon, 224
Knee arthritis, 19–21, 197–198
Koop, Everett, 11

Laetrile, 69
Landau, Bill, 232–233, 235
Landau, Reuben, 232–233, 235
Laparoscopy, 47–48
Larynx cancer, 43–44
Lasell College/Lasell Village, 247
Laser eye surgery, 120–121
Lavage and debridement, 20–21
Leukemia, 119
Lewy Body disease, 8
Life, prolongation of, 43–44, 46, 48, 64–69, 72–73, 76, 81, 85, 114–115, 259
Life cycle, 209, 220–222
Life expectancy, 5, 26, 32–33, 45, 206, 211–212, 218–220
Life experiences, 230, 247
Life Line monitor, 171
Liposuction, 4, 219
Live-in assistants, 2
London, 89–90
Longevity, 3–4, 203, 205–214, 218–224, 284–285
Lumpectomy, 61
Lung disorders: pneumonia, 7, 45, 64–66, 72, 75, 118; pulmonary embolism, 22, 96; emphysema, 56, 114

Lung volume reduction surgery, 114, 120

MacArthur Foundation Study of Successful Aging, 235
Macular degeneration, 7, 56
Mammograms, 11, 17, 27, 30, 32, 111, 258. *See also* Breast cancer
Marriott, 179–180
Massachusetts General Hospital, 28
Massachusetts Institute of Technology, 275
Mastectomy, 61
McGowan Institute for Regenerative Medicine, 285
Medicaid, 106–108, 112–113, 119, 121, 137, 149–150, 155, 157, 167, 182, 188–191, 219, 275
Medicare, 5, 7, 9, 21, 30, 46, 57, 61, 81–82, 103–106, 214, 219, 275, 279–280; and prescription drugs, 93, 98, 156; and nursing homes, 93, 98–103, 106–110, 113, 125, 137, 149–150, 155–156; good/bad aspects of program, 93–94, 119–121; and hospitalization, 94, 96–103, 109–110, 113, 115, 120; and home care, 96–103, 106–108; and hospices, 102–103, 110–111; proposed three-plan system, 111–119; and assisted living, 178, 188–191, 193; need to reform, 255–256, 260–263, 265
Medicare Advantage, 116
Medicare plus Choice, 116
Medicare Prescription Drug Improvement and Modernization Act, 93, 98, 156, 280
Medicare Rights Center, 279–280
Medication: prescription drugs, 9, 35, 88, 93, 111, 116, 156, 163, 183–185, 261; taking, 127, 163, 184–185

MediGap policies, 116, 261
Metchnikoff, Elie, 223
Miller, Richard, 206
Milwaukee, Wis., 180
Minimum Data Set, 146, 148, 150–151
Minneapolis, Minn., 70
Minnesota, 168–169, 188
Missionary work, 244
Mobility, 139–140, 248
Modern Maturity, 5
Morphine, 53–55, 64, 66
Moses, Grandma (Anna Mary Robertson), 234–235
Multiple myeloma, 238

National Center for Assisted Living, 283
National Center on Caregiving, 277
National Citizens' Coalition for Nursing Home Reform, 145–146, 156, 181, 281
National Commission for the Protection of Human Subjects of Biomedical and Behavioral Research, 79–80
National Conference of Catholic Bishops, 66–67
National Family Caregiver Support Program, 154
National Hospice and Palliative Care Organization, 278
National Institutes of Health, 82, 121
National Public Radio, 233–234
National Senior Citizens' Law Center, 181
Nausea, 37–39
Nazis, 227–229
Negotiated risk contracts, 185–188
New England Centenarian Study, 211–212, 284
New England Journal of Medicine, 21, 252, 264
New urbanism, 244–245

New York, 178, 187
New York Times, 232–233
New York University, 229–231
Nuland, Sherwin: *How We Die,* 256
Nurse practitioners, 59–61, 101–102
Nurses, 58–60, 87, 97–98, 101, 127, 129, 132, 147, 163–164, 184
Nursing aides, 128–134, 143, 145, 147, 152–154, 183
Nursing Home Compare, 137, 139–141, 281
Nursing Home Reform Act, 146
Nursing homes, 2, 9, 41, 44, 46, 60, 66, 74, 124–131, 137–144, 159–160, 164, 167, 170, 178, 181–182, 190–192, 200, 214, 281–282; and Medicare/Medicaid, 93, 98–103, 106–110, 112–113, 119, 121, 125, 137, 149–150, 155–156; number of residents, 123–124, 152–153; caregivers in, 127–134, 145, 147, 151–155; quality of care/life, 131–133, 137, 139, 149–150; model, 131–137; shopping for, 137, 139–141; regulation of, 144–148; need to reform, 148–157, 255, 262–263; growing need for facilities, 151–153
Nutrition. *See* Diet

Obesity, 209, 257–258
Okinawans, 212–213
Old age homes, 164–167
Omnibus Reconciliation Act, 146
On Lok Senior Health Services, 112
Oregon, 83, 91, 121
Orthopedic surgery, 19–21
Oshkosh, Wis., 170
Osteoarthritis, 7, 19–21, 197–198
Osteoporosis, 22, 35, 111, 121, 215–216
Overpopulation, 218
Overtreatment, 37, 63
Oxygen, 50, 64–66, 238

Pacemakers, 198–199
Palliative care, 94, 103, 111, 114–119, 253, 259, 277–279
Pap smear tests, 17, 31, 259. *See also* Cervical cancer
Parkinson's disease, 33, 106
Partnership for Solutions, 276
Peripheral vascular disease, 56
Perls, Tom, 211–212
Personal care attendants, 153–154
Peru, 155
Phenobarbital, 83
Philippines, 155
Physical examinations, 15–19, 23, 26, 32, 36
Physical therapy, 54–55, 139, 216
Physician assistants, 59
Physician-assisted suicide, 83, 88, 91, 252–253
Pick's disease, 8
Pioneer Network, 133–134, 136, 281–282
Pittsburgh Medical Center, 285
Planned communities, 244–245, 247–248
Plastic surgery, 119
Platter-Zyberk, Elizabeth, 244
Pneumonia, 7, 45, 64–66, 72, 75, 118
Podiatry, 113, 169
Political activism, 256–257, 266
Ponce de León, Juan, 223
Poorhouses, 166
Preferences, treatment, 8, 43–48, 60
Prescription drugs, 9, 35, 88, 93, 111, 116, 156, 163, 183–185, 261
President's Council on Bioethics, 220–221, 224
Pressure ulcers, 142, 146, 178
Preventive health. *See* Annual checkups; Screening tests
Preventive Services Task Force, 16–17, 81, 274

Progesterone, 22

Program of All-Inclusive Care for the Elderly, 110–114, 275–276

Prolongation of life. *See* Life, prolongation of

Prostate cancer, 12–17, 24–27, 29, 33–34

Prostatectomy, 24–25

Prostate specific antigen (PSA) test, 12–17, 26–27, 33–34, 111, 258–259

Protestantism/Protestants, 165

Providence Mount Saint Vincent, 132–133, 135

Proxies. *See* Health care proxies

Public health departments, state, 144–146, 149, 178–179

Pulmonary embolism, 22, 96

Puritans, 4, 221–222

Putnam, Robert: *Bowling Alone*, 250–251

Quality of care, 137, 178, 180, 182–183, 192, 214

Quality of life, 10, 12, 19, 48, 131–133, 139, 149–150, 181, 205, 259, 262–263, 265

Radiology, 27–29

Radiotherapy, 43–44, 115

Recreation therapy, 131, 147, 150

Regent Assisted Living, 179

Rejuvenon, 195

Rest homes, 164–167

Restraints, 141, 146

Retirement, 5, 226–232, 238–244, 285–287; making most of, 225–226; model retirees, 232–235; self-fulfillment programs, 235–238; communities, 244–250; and autonomy, 250–253

Retirement Living Information Center, 285–286

Retirement Research Foundation, 286–287

Robertson, Anna Mary (Grandma Moses), 234–235

Robert Wood Johnson Foundation, 112, 276

Rochester, N. Y., 136

Roxbury Home for Aged Women, 166

Russia, 5

St. Christopher's Hospice, 89–90

St. Joseph's Irish Sisters of Charity Hospital, 90

San Diego, Calif., 16

Saunders, Cicely, 89–90

Schorr, Daniel, 233–235

Screening tests, 6, 14–19, 26–34, 36, 82, 111, 258–259. *See also specific tests*

Seaside, Fla., 244–245

Seattle, Wash., 132, 136

Sickle cell anemia, 118, 207–208

Sigmoidoscopy, 17

Skin cancer, 196–197

Sleeping pills, 127

Smoking, 11, 36, 56

Social contacts, 258–259

Social Security, 5, 125, 188

Special Committee on Aging (Senate), 3, 180

Stem cells, 209

Steroids, 87

Stroke, 1–3, 22, 30–31, 36, 57–58, 106, 257–258

Struldbruggs, 204–205

Study to Understand Prognoses and Preferences for Care, 43, 60

Suburban life, 244–245, 263

Suffering, 65–68, 75

Suicide, 83, 88, 91, 252–253

Sun City, 226

Superoxide dismutase, 210
Supplemental Social Security Insurance, 188
Surgeon-General, Office of the, 11
Surgery, 19–21, 42–44, 47–48, 119
Surrogates. *See* Health care proxies
Surveyors, state, 144–146
Swift, Jonathan, 204–205
Switzerland, 228–229

Tai chi, 35
Talmud, 68
Task Force on the Periodic Health Examination (Canada), 16, 81
Tasma, David, 89
Television shows, 264–266
Telomeres/telomerase, 208, 210
Tests. *See* Screening tests
Texas, 78–79
Thomas, Bill, 134–136, 151
Thomas, Judy, 134–135
Thrombosis, 22, 96–98
Time, 168
Tithonus myth, 203–205
Total institutions, 128–129
Treatment preferences, 8, 43–48, 60
Tumors, 85–88. *See also* Cancer
Tutoring, 231, 237–238, 286

University of California, 234
University of Minnesota, 150

University of North Carolina at Asheville, 246–247
University of Pittsburgh, 285
Urban life, 244–245, 263
Urinary tract infection, 39–40
Uterine cancer, 22

Vaillant, George, 268
Vascular dementia, 7
Vegetative state, 73–74, 78
Ventilators, 70–71
Veterans Administration, 106
Virtual communities, 248–250
Vitamins, 3; B12, 198; E, 210; D, 216
Volunteer work, 231–232, 236–238, 247, 250, 286
Vomiting, 37–38

Wanglie, Helga, 70–71
Warfarin, 58–59
Weight control, 209, 257–259, 261–262
Wellsprings, 154
West, Michael, 208–209
Winfrey, Oprah, 28–29
Wolfe, Alan, 250
Women's Health Initiative, 22

X-rays, 27, 49

Yankelovich, Daniel, 250